Fight Heart Disease
Like Cancer

Fight Heart Disease Like Cancer

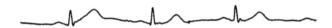

Michael V. McConnell, MD, MSEE

Johns Hopkins University Press | Baltimore

© 2024 Johns Hopkins University Press
All rights reserved. Published 2024
Printed in the United States of America on acid-free paper
9   8   7   6   5   4   3   2   1

Johns Hopkins University Press
2715 North Charles Street
Baltimore, Maryland 21218
www.press.jhu.edu

Library of Congress Cataloging-in-Publication Data is available.

A catalog record for this book is available from the British Library.

ISBN 978-1-4214-4846-6 (hardcover)
ISBN 978-1-4214-4848-0 (ebook)

Special discounts are available for bulk purchases of this book. For more information, please contact Special Sales at specialsales@jh.edu.

To the strong, amazing women in my family who've inspired and supported me—Jane, Lily, Patrice, Alicia, Kelly, Mia, and especially Lena. All my love and gratitude.

Contents

Fight Heart Disease
Like Cancer

Introduction

If you had a choice, would you want your doctor to diagnose you with heart disease or cancer? My guess is heart disease, even though it can kill in minutes, often without warning, and it kills more people in the United States and around the world than cancer. But if I asked how you'd like to be treated once diagnosed, you'd likely say cancer, for the high level of concern, care, and caring from family, friends, and health care providers.

As a preventive cardiologist, my hope in writing this book is simple—to help stop people from dying of heart disease. To do this, we must start treating it more like cancer at every level: from the understanding that heart disease—like a cancerous tumor—can grow silently within us, to the importance of screening to detect early disease before it's "malignant," to the use of modern therapy to turn heart disease from malignant to benign.

What if I told you that heart disease and cancer share five risk factors, and the original medical term for heart disease was "tumor"? What if I told you that there's a heart disease gene as lethal as the breast cancer gene *BRCA* that's easier to test for and treat, but 80% of people don't know they have it? What if I told you that there's a heart screening test like a mammogram that can detect early disease but is rarely used, and that mammograms themselves can detect early heart disease in women but this information isn't included in the results? What if I told you that there's safe and powerful "chemotherapy" to reverse heart disease, with the newest therapy taken only twice per year? And is every man over 50 and woman over 60 you know on preventive therapy, or do they have a negative screening test?

As you can tell from my questions, there are major similarities between heart disease and cancer that provide opportunities for us to fight heart disease more effectively. You can probably also tell I'm frustrated that heart disease care hasn't caught up to cancer care. We haven't done a good enough job educating our patients, or our health care colleagues, about these important similarities, which could dramatically improve the three pillars of heart disease care—prevention, screening, and treatment—and stop heart disease in its tracks for all.

I hope you'll join me on a journey of discovery, and sometimes rediscovery, to learn how heart disease and cancer are intertwined, not only scientifically but personally. These diseases impact our lives and those of family and friends, and also made people more vulnerable to the ravages of the recent COVID-19 pandemic. I want to give you information to help you better understand heart disease and how to help yourself and your loved ones avoid its dire consequences. My drive to reach as many people as I can stems from how I've seen heart disease and cancer affect me, my family, and my patients. In my career as a scientist and preventive cardiologist, I've learned that it's important to think more like an oncologist (a cancer specialist) in both research and clinical care.

It always starts with family. Our family was devastated when my father-in-law died suddenly of a heart attack—"on my watch." What did I learn from that and what can you? There would be even more heart disease on my wife's side of the family and multiple cancers on mine, leading us to consider the risks to our daughters. At the same time, my medical and research career has evolved from developing technologies at Harvard and Stanford to see inside the heart to detect early disease to then working on digital health initiatives with Apple, Google, and Fitbit to promote prevention for millions (even billions) of people across the world. Along the way, my colleagues and I were discovering, or rediscovering, the many similarities between heart disease and cancer. Yet this information, despite all the review articles in medical journals, isn't getting to patients and their health care providers. As with cancer, preventing and treating heart disease is more about stopping "tumors" from growing than fixing our "plumbing." Gaining this perspective from family and career experiences has changed my approach to patients, as you'll read in the next chapter. I hope you'll take this new approach— of fighting heart disease like cancer—to help yourself and your loved ones.

Note: In addition to the references provided throughout and listed at the end of the book, there are short URLs/links included in the text for easy access to videos, interviews, blog posts, and heart health guides (under "FHDLC.info").

CHAPTER 1

Straight Talk

Heart Disease Is Like Cancer,
Only Worse

Blunt Language

"You basically have cancer in your heart arteries." The first time I said this to a patient, they broke out in a cold sweat.

I'm a cardiologist, not an oncologist, so why did I say that and why do I continue to say it to my patients? They need to hear straight talk from me if we're going to work together to prevent them from dying too young from heart disease. This had become personal as well as professional for me. I'd seen heart disease and cancer in my family, and my research was showing increasing similarities between the two killers. I needed to help my patients understand what I'd learned through my life and career—that we need to fight heart disease like cancer.

In medical school, we learn how to take a good patient history, perform a detailed physical exam, and establish a diagnosis and treatment plan. For my patient, like many in my clinic, a scan showed calcium deposits in the blood vessels that supply the heart. This meant that there was *plaque*, originally called a fatty "tumor," growing inside the heart. This is the main form of heart disease that causes heart attacks. Although we had made the diagnosis and started preventive medication to keep the plaque from growing, the patient stopped taking it. For me, it was like an oncologist hearing their cancer patient had stopped chemotherapy.

What we're not taught so well is how to communicate effectively what we know (and don't know) and what we recommend to our patients. Clearly, I didn't communicate the seriousness of the diagnosis effectively with my patient. I knew from my research and the recent loss of my father-in-law to a sudden heart attack that, left untreated, my patient's heart disease could become "malignant." Worse than a malignant cancer, it could cause a heart attack and kill them in minutes. Many colleagues and I were finding increasing similarities between heart disease and cancer, from underlying biology to imaging to treatment. Telling a patient they had the equivalent of cancer in their heart arteries was not only straight talk to help them take the diagnosis seriously—it matched the latest science.

I'd like to say that this message has gotten out to more patients and physicians, but it hasn't. In medical journals, there are more articles every year on the overlap between heart disease and cancer, but this information is stuck there. Telling patients and their families one at a time does not spread the message. In this social media world, there are blog posts, tweets, TED talks, and so on to get information into the world, but I'm starting with this book to help spread this lifesaving message to all. My goal is to use the journeys of my family, my patients, and my scientific career to help you and your loved ones (and even your doctor) understand and *fight heart disease like cancer*—from prevention to screening to therapy. Let me help you keep heart disease benign and avoid what happened to my father-in-law.

A Tragic Missed Opportunity on My Watch

James Wu was born in Hong Kong and met my mother-in-law, Lily, when they were students in Taiwan. Like many of their generation, they came to the United States as graduate students and stayed to start careers and raise a family. They became professors at the University of Utah. As fate would have it, James was an expert on early markers of disease, especially cancer. One of his earliest publications was in the *New England*

Journal of Medicine on the use of blood tests to monitor cancer.[1] He went on to write multiple books on the decades of progress that followed in the development of *circulating tumor markers*, which have become the mainstay of cancer care (including for my sister, as we'll learn later). When we met, James had started turning his tumor marker expertise toward the study of circulating heart disease markers. During my cardiology fellowship in Boston, I introduced him to colleagues studying a blood marker common to both heart disease and cancer.[2,3] As we'll discuss, Lily was an expert in cholesterol testing. Together, James and Lily wrote an article on all the emerging blood tests for early detection of heart disease.[4] Their words were accurate and prescient as they highlighted the importance of prevention and early detection: "detecting early risk markers" for heart disease is important "to avoid serious or fatal consequences." Unfortunately, James didn't apply what he studied in the lab to his own health.

In general, my father-in-law and I got along well. He liked that his son-in-law was a doctor and an engineer and we enjoyed discussing his research. He spoiled my two daughters—as grandparents will do. Where we did not get along well was around his own health. It was clear, from his busy work and travel schedule, that he wasn't making time for physical activity or following a healthy diet. While he liked discussing science with doctors, he didn't want to see one. I heard, through Lily, that he periodically had to slow down when walking and had symptoms of diabetes, but my attempts to encourage him to improve his lifestyle and see a doctor fell on deaf ears.

Almost every winter, I'd bring my daughters, Kelly and Mia, to visit James and Lily in Salt Lake City as a dad-daughter and grandparent-granddaughter trip. I vividly recall arguing with James on one of these trips in front of Lily and my daughters. We all went out for a meal and he intentionally ordered the unhealthiest items on the menu, loaded with meat and carbohydrates. Of course, I couldn't stay silent and made my anger known. I knew how much Kelly and Mia, sitting right there, loved him and how much he loved them. It was not just about getting healthy for himself or me. It was about being there for Kelly and Mia and watching them grow up.

It was only a few years later when we got that fateful call. He was in Taiwan, advising a large hospital there. He'd given a lecture and then was taken out to a celebratory meal. The entourage took a van back from dinner. When it arrived, he didn't get up from his seat. He died in transit, just like that. A heart attack stopped his heart from supplying the blood and oxygen his body needed to function. It's like the power going out, but it can't be turned on later and go back to normal. He was gone.

Our family was devastated. Mia and Kelly were only 9 and 12 at the time. We all went to Taiwan for the funeral and met many extended family members. At one of the family gatherings, the natural question came up—how did he have a heart attack when his son-in-law was a Stanford cardiologist? That was a hard question to hear, but I was already asking it myself. He died of heart disease on my watch. I had tried to communicate my concerns, but they clearly didn't get through. I ask myself: What if he understood how important he was to my family and daughters? What if Kelly and Mia were old enough at the time to understand the connection and pleaded with him? What if I communicated more effectively how serious heart disease could be? It was clearly worse than cancer in his case, taking him so quickly we couldn't say goodbye. This event started me on my journey to approach prevention better. We needed better science around early detection but also better ways to fight heart disease like cancer. Maybe if he could see all the similarities that are now being published, he'd have found the connection in his own research with a bit more time.

Granddaughters' Wishes

My daughters have been part of the inspiration for writing this book. Partly, this is because of the sudden loss of their grandfather. More so, it's because they can share the perspective of a child or grandchild wanting their parents or grandparents alive and healthy—to be there for graduations, weddings, careers, and families. Wise words from a cardiologist like me can help, but people are often most compelled to act when it's to help those around them. Plus, it's my daughters' generation that can incorporate these ideas and help turn heart disease benign.

Mia was only 9 when her grandfather died and wished she'd known how to change his fate.

Waking up one morning and having my parents tell me that you had died from a heart attack was one of the hardest things I've had to go through. For weeks I couldn't stop thinking about you. Thinking that I would never get to see you, hold your hand, or hear your voice ever again. The last time I said goodbye to you I was only thinking goodbye for a few months, not forever. I told you I loved you, but I thought I would be telling you I loved you for many more years to come. I know you didn't choose to pass away early and suddenly but I still wish you could've been around to see Kelly and I grow up. I also wish that I could have known more about your health and known more about how to help you so I could have at least tried to keep you around longer.

Kelly was 12 and already interested in how the heart worked and what her dad did as a cardiologist. But she'd witnessed that science isn't enough. We need to teach and help each other, and she realized that a book like this could be part of that.

So why should you, the reader, continue reading the book? I could go on and list facts, about heart disease is the #1 cause of death in the U.S. but that isn't relevant. You should keep reading so that you can make a difference in a life, whether it be your own or someone else's; So you can prevent a grandparent, parent, aunt, uncle, friend from dying suddenly, leaving too early from your life.

Now Mia and Kelly are grown, having graduated from college and embarked on their own careers. The pain of their grandfather's death may be less acute, but their perspective on wanting those around them, and their world, to be healthier for all has matured. They've also seen more cardiovascular disease on my wife, Lena's, side of the family and cancer on mine. Fortunately, we know to take both seriously and are still around for them. We want the same for you and your loved ones.

CHAPTER 2

How Did We Get Here?

The Twin Pandemics of Heart Disease and Cancer

Throughout most of known human history, infectious diseases have been the great killers. We've experienced this again with the COVID-19 pandemic that caused close to seven million deaths worldwide from early 2020 through 2022.[5] But for perspective, heart disease caused eight times as many deaths over the same period—it kills 19 million people worldwide every year! Cancer killed over four times as many people as COVID-19 over this period at 10 million per year.[6,7] Thus, the real "pandemics" of the last century have been the marked rise of these noninfectious diseases as the leading killers. You'll also hear them referred to as "noncommunicable diseases," or NCDs. As we'll discuss, science is showing the many ways in which they're intertwined beyond "competing" to be most lethal. Indeed, my colleagues and I highlighted the need to move beyond approaching them separately in our American Heart Association's (AHA) 2030 Impact Goal report. We and the AHA called for a new, comprehensive, and equitable approach to heart disease *and* cancer prevention if we're all to live in a healthy and productive world.[8]

The Rise and Fall and Rise of Heart Disease

The story of the rise of heart disease and our efforts against it is clearly one of great progress initially, but it's now one of unfinished business and even reversal. In 1900, heart disease was the number four killer after pneumonia/influenza, tuberculosis (TB), and intestinal infections.[9] With improvements in public health and antibiotics, infectious diseases declined such that every year since the influenza pandemic of 1918–1920, heart disease has been number one. By the 1940s, heart disease and stroke (together called *cardiovascular disease*) were causing half—yes, half!—of all deaths in the United States. Despite this, it took a president's death to spur action.

As the longest-serving US president, Franklin D. Roosevelt is known for many things. One thing most people don't realize is his impact on the understanding and prevention of heart disease. Over his 12-year presidency spanning the Great Depression to World War II, he became progressively weaker, while his blood pressure went from just above normal to what we'd now call a *hypertensive crisis*. (Later, we'll go into more detail about high blood pressure as a big contributor to heart disease.) Yet FDR's doctors ascribed his sky-high blood pressure to "normal aging," based on what they knew at the time. It was his daughter Anna who insisted he see a cardiologist, who diagnosed him with heart failure and helped with the limited treatments of the time. It ultimately took Winston Churchill's physician to make the main diagnosis—"hardening of the arteries"—and predict that he only had a few months to live. It was still a surprise to his American doctors when FDR died suddenly from a stroke only a few weeks later with a blood pressure almost three times normal!

From this came a national effort to understand cardiovascular disease (referred to at the time as "diseases of the heart and circulation") to stem this new "pandemic." FDR's successor, Harry Truman, signed the National Heart Act, establishing the National Heart Institute for research within the National Institutes of Health (NIH). He also provided the initial funding for what became the Framingham Heart Study.

Framingham, the Start of Our Understanding of Heart Disease

In the 1940s, Framingham, Massachusetts, was a town of 28,000 and typical of the US population at the time. It was also close to Boston and the cardiologists affiliated with Harvard Medical School, who would oversee the study. Framingham residents had previously participated in a study of tuberculosis and agreed to this new study of heart disease.

While revolutionary at the time, the study's concept was simple: collect as much health-related data as possible and observe who developed heart disease and which measured factors contributed to it. Unlike infectious disease, where a single virus or bacterium is the cause, researchers found many different factors contributed to heart disease. Indeed, the concept of multiple *risk factors* came from the Framingham study. Many are likely familiar—blood cholesterol, blood pressure, and blood glucose, as well as cigarette smoking, obesity, and sedentary lifestyle. So much was learned from the people of Framingham. They continue to contribute to our understandings today because the study continues 70 years later and includes the grandchildren of the original participants.[10,11]

Importantly, the lessons of Framingham were applied through national campaigns to combat high cholesterol, high blood pressure, and cigarette smoking. Great progress was made over the next 30 years. The NIH had experts convene at its headquarters in Bethesda, Maryland in the late 1970s to understand why heart disease had declined so profoundly to become number two, behind cancer, in some analyses of the statistics. While this was a great achievement, these experts recognized that there was much left to do. Unfortunately, this has taken on more urgency because the prior downward "bending of the curve" for heart disease deaths each decade stopped at the end of the 20th century. In the 21st century, we've seen a re-rise in heart disease spreading across the globe, so the curve has bent upward again. I had the privilege of participating in a reconvening of experts by the AHA in 2018 to review these disturbing trends. Recognizing that there's a lot left to do, we presented a range of emerging opportunities—several included in this book—to bend the curve back downward.[12]

How Did We Get to This Point, with All That We Know?

There are many reasons we're seeing the re-rise of heart disease, including the obesity epidemic and rise in diabetes; the ongoing inequity in access to quality care; and the short and long-term exacerbation of heart disease by COVID-19. But I've become convinced that the major reason is that we're not approaching heart disease care like we approach cancer care, even though we keep learning more about how these diseases are intertwined.

How did we get to this point where, despite all the scientific evidence, we don't treat heart disease as seriously as we should? I'm not a psychologist, so I'm not an expert on what people think, but I can tell you what I've seen over many years. The major reason, and theme in this book, is that we continue to think of heart disease as a simple problem of clogged pipes that need opening. Rather, it's much more like a growing tumor in the heart vessels that can become malignant and needs serious care—and straight talk—to be stopped.

Ironically, I started out as an engineer. Part of my interest in cardiology was that heart disease, even among cardiologists, was viewed as an engineering problem, from clogged vessels limiting blood flow, to the heart muscle struggling to pump, to the heart's electrical activity going awry—the same sequence of events that caused James Wu's heart to stop. Little did I realize that I'd learn and advocate to treat heart disease more like an oncologist than an engineer.

There are certainly engineering aspects of heart disease treatment. We have mechanical ways to deal with clogged arteries, such as balloons, stents, and surgery, but they make it seem like we can "fix" heart disease. If we don't stop the biology, however, the malignant growth will continue and cause a heart attack in a different place in our "pipes" that we didn't fix. Similarly, for most cancers, surgery can remove the bulk of the tumor, but it can grow back from malignant cells we can't remove. That's why chemotherapy is often used after surgery to attack the biology and prevent the cancer from coming back. This is one example of where learning from cancer care can apply to heart disease care.

Another reason I alluded to is complacency. The better job we've done explaining and treating heart disease as an engineering problem, the less fearful it seems and the more complacent patients and physicians become. I don't know how many times I've been told by patients, or read in the newspaper, about a "perfectly healthy" person felled by heart disease "out of the blue." I remind them that this is actually very common. Less than 10% of adults in the United States have optimal heart health.[13] Women understandably worry about breast cancer, but often don't realize that heart attack deaths among women are four times more common than breast cancer deaths in the United States.[14] While most know that heart disease can occur earlier in men, few realize that one in two get heart disease in their lifetime despite all the progress we've made, compared to less than one in twenty who get colon cancer.[15,16] Shockingly, when I talk with friends my age who are at the prime "at risk" time in their lives for having their life cut short by heart disease, many haven't had screening and preventive therapy conversations with their physicians. Yet they continue to diligently get their mammograms and colonoscopies. Go figure.

A third reason is another positive with unanticipated consequences. We've shown that heart disease is preventable with healthy behaviors, which makes it seem like it's easier to prevent and treat than cancer. Like the patient I introduced the book with, there's a perception that a bit more physical activity and a better diet can completely take care of it. As a preventive cardiologist, I wholeheartedly support patients' efforts to prevent heart disease through a healthy lifestyle. I'm also realistic, however, and believe in the scientific evidence that healthy behaviors alone may not be enough for everyone. Therefore, screening for early disease and using medication when needed to stop it from growing and killing are as important in cardiology as they are in oncology. We know exercise and a healthy diet can help prevent many cancers, but that doesn't stop us from needing regular cancer screening and effective therapies.

The final reason, and another major stimulus for writing this book, is that most people, even health care providers, are behind on the latest science on the similarities between heart disease and cancer and the resulting opportunities to improve care. I believe that increasing this awareness among patients and providers can enhance our ability to fight heart disease, from prevention to screening to treatment. Ironically, when the main cause of heart attacks was noted, hundreds of years ago, to be from abnormal tissue growth in the heart, it was given the name *atheroma*, based on the Greek word for tumor. We're overdue to understand again that heart disease is from malignant tumors that can be as devastating as the worst cancers. Further, discoveries in cancer diagnosis and treatment offer new ways to treat heart disease. This isn't the science of the future; rather, it's the science of today and is published extensively. Our health care system has been slow to follow the science and we practitioners have been slow to educate our patients. Maybe this book can empower you to call for the end of heart disease as cancer patients have lobbied to end cancer. Just like cancer patients, you deserve the best care based on the best science.

CHAPTER 3

Learning from Cancer in My Family and Myself

My Early Career Misconceptions

My daughters losing their grandfather to heart disease crystalized my desire to prevent that from happening to others. My own grandfather's life and death also have an important place in this story. His life inspired my career, but his death contributed to my early misconceptions about heart disease and cancer. James Carroll grew up in New York City during the Depression and earned an engineering degree from Cooper Union College while working a full-time job. He worked his way up through the New York City government, retiring after 40 years as part of a generation of Irish civil servants the *New York Times* tongue-in-cheek called the "Irish Mafia."[17] I have great memories of him taking me to catch blowfish on Long Island. He inspired me to go to MIT to become an engineer like him.

The summer before senior year at MIT was my introduction to biomedical engineering and heart disease. I did an internship at Medtronic in Minneapolis, the first company to make an implantable pacemaker. The idea that a device could be programmed to deliver a small amount of electricity to make the heart beat every second of every day for years thrilled the engineer in me. I wanted to learn about the heart and do more to treat it. That inspired my thesis research when I went back to MIT for my senior year, but my grandfather wouldn't be there to see me graduate. That December, he was diagnosed with advanced stomach cancer. I loved my grandfather deeply, and I was crushed that he was taken from us on the cusp of my graduating in his footsteps.

Looking back, I realize that this initial personal experience of heart disease and cancer matched the conventional understanding of these diseases for most of the 20th century. Heart disease is often viewed as an engineering problem—a pump that may need new wiring, valves, or plumbing to improve blood supply. Cancer, on the other hand, is seen as a mysterious growth requiring surgery to remove and chemicals to kill, often unsuccessfully. Heart disease sounds more "fixable." Cancer, more deadly.

As an engineer, I naturally gravitated toward working on heart disease. Thus, my journey to become a cardiologist began. As you'll learn, I had to go beyond engineering in my research and care of patients to apply principles of cancer science and care to the study and treatment of heart disease.

Cancer Gets Personal

"It looks like it could be cancer." "I need to do a biopsy." "Are you going to be OK?" These aren't words anyone wants to hear, including me. It was only two years after my father-in-law died. My wife losing her father and my daughters losing their grandfather was terrible, but having them lose a husband and father soon after would be devastating. I was concerned, but OK, and not too surprised. I had made the appointment to get checked. I have fair Irish skin, and when I grew up, the strong sunscreen we have now didn't exist. We had "suntan" lotion back then, and there wasn't much emphasis on sun protection. I had a few benign skin growths at this point, but I knew my father had several small skin cancers removed. What really got me to make another dermatology appointment was my sister telling me she may have skin cancer.

I could hear the concern in my dermatologist's voice as she looked at a spot on my back. She asked if I thought the spot had been getting bigger. I had no clue—it was in the middle of my upper back, an area I never see in the mirror. I told her she should not hold back and tell me what she thought. If I can use cancer terminology when I talk with patients about their heart disease, she should be frank when it comes to cancer itself. She thought it was melanoma—there's that "-oma" term again, meaning tumor. Worse, the full name for this skin cancer is *malignant melanoma*, leaving no room for doubt about its seriousness.

When my grandfather died of cancer while I was in college, it all happened so quickly that I didn't appreciate all the care and family involvement that goes into cancer diagnosis and treatment. Now that I likely had it, I could experience, firsthand, a different health care journey. Even that first conversation with my dermatologist, with her careful way of expressing her presumed diagnosis, even to another doctor, revealed a lot. She knew from experience that any mention of cancer raises the specter of a life-ending disease. This also helped me realize that I'd been more casual about telling patients they have plaque "tumors" in their heart arteries than my dermatologist was in telling me I had skin cancer.

A biopsy and pathology report revealed that it was indeed malignant melanoma. Thankfully, it hadn't grown very deep, and the prognosis was good. She reviewed the risks and recommended surgery alone without chemotherapy. That surgery was over 10 years ago and there's been no recurrence. My sister also had an early melanoma with successful surgery. We both dodged a bullet and were appreciative of the attentive care we received. Personally and professionally, I could see the comprehensive care that goes into cancer treatment and the strong support from family and friends. Deservedly so. It makes a big difference.

More Cancer Strikes

The real shock to our family was when my sister developed a more serious form of cancer than the malignant melanoma we'd shared. She started feeling discomfort in the upper stomach area, where the liver and gallbladder are. Imaging showed tumors near her liver and ovaries. She had Stage 3 ovarian cancer. It started in her ovaries but spread silently without symptoms until it formed a big enough growth to hurt her liver.

This was a devastating diagnosis for her, her husband, her three children, our family, and her multitude of friends. Jumping ahead, she's had amazing care and support and continues to keep her cancer at bay. Her experience is where our family learned what modern cancer care can and should be for all. It's a team effort that starts on the medical side, where oncologists and surgeons work together on options, informed further by pathologists' review of the cancer cell biology. This leads to a shared decision with patients on treatment plans, which can be a combination of surgery, chemotherapy, or radiation. Then there are the friends and family who rally around to support trips for surgery, lab testing, and chemotherapy and the great nurses who work with patients along the journey.

Key to my sister's success is how cancer care has evolved to recognize that it's not always as simple as my skin cancer, where surgical removal can be the cure. Instead, a combination of surgery, chemotherapy, and even newer forms of growth inhibitors can keep a cancer mostly dormant. Regular checks to see if it's started to reemerge can guide escalating therapy to keep it at bay. In many ways, this aspect of cancer care is evolving to be more like heart disease care, where the focus is on lifelong care to prevent heart attacks. Our approach to fighting heart disease really needs to learn from how seriously cancer is treated and how every tool in the armamentarium is used—from careful blood monitoring to imaging for tumor growth to escalating treatment when growth is found. Also, there's more understanding when talking with patients and their families about upcoming challenges and risks and more involvement of family and friends in supporting them through the process.

CHAPTER 4

Understanding Your Heart and Its Vulnerability

An Ever-Beating Pump

Before we dive too far into the details of how heart disease and cancer overlap, it's important to understand the basics of how the heart works and where heart disease starts. I've taught how the heart works throughout my career, starting when I was a biomedical engineering teaching assistant at MIT. I still find it amazing. The heart is a muscle whose job is to pump blood throughout the body like how a central pumping station provides water to a city, an engine powers a car, or a generator provides electricity to a town. Unlike the muscles in your arms or legs that contract when you tell them, the heart contracts on its own. That makes sense because unlike an engine or generator, you can't just turn the heart off. If the heart stops, the blood supply to the whole body stops, and then we stop.

This amazing feature—that heart muscle cells beat on their own—starts early in fetal life. If you grow heart cells in a petri dish, they will start to beat together. Each heart cell has an electrical "timer" that triggers its muscle fibers to contract repeatedly. When one cell beats, it passes that electrical trigger to the next, telling it to beat. This allows the heart to pump in a coordinated fashion every second of every day to keep us alive.

The heart has four chambers with a right and left side. The upper chambers are the *atria*, and they collect blood returning to the heart. The lower chambers are the *ventricles*, and they do the harder part of pumping the blood out of the heart. The right ventricle pumps blood to the lungs for oxygen and the left ventricle pumps the oxygenated blood to the rest of the body. There are also one-way valves to make sure blood is pumped forward (Figure 4.1).

It may seem hard to believe, but it took thousands of years for medicine to understand how the heart worked. Early on, they realized that both sides of the heart moved blood around the body, but they couldn't figure out how the blood went from the right side of the heart to the left. They couldn't see, with the naked eye, how the blood vessels keep branching into smaller vessels until they become *capillaries*, which need a microscope to see. Eventually, they understood that blood circulated from *arteries* (vessels that leave the heart) into capillaries and then into *veins* (vessels that return to the heart). Thus, the single artery that leaves the left ventricle—the *aorta*—branches into billions of capillaries so that every part of the body gets blood to deliver oxygen and nutrients. Per our earlier analogy, the heart is the central pump or power station, but it needs a network of pipes to deliver water to every home.

The main form of heart disease starts in these pipes—the arteries. This discovery was made by a scientist who combined engineering and medicine (and art!)—Leonardo da Vinci. While he's famous for painting the Mona Lisa that hangs in the Louvre, he's also famous for his human anatomy drawings—and doing engineering experiments to understand how parts of the body worked. He had a healthy medical curiosity, which led to his discovery of the main form of heart disease. It started when he met an old man who described his good fortune to feel well without any limiting symptoms of old age. But several hours later, da Vinci heard the man had died, without visible cause, eerily like my father-in-law. Da Vinci was among a select few allowed to do autopsies at the time. He found thickened artery walls and concluded that the man

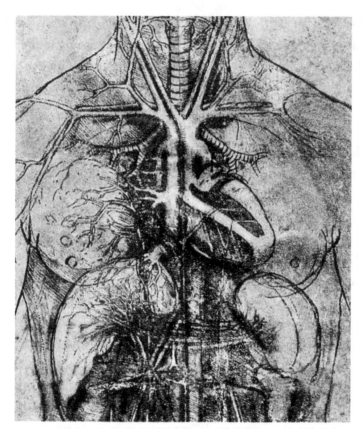

FIGURE 4.1   Anatomic drawing of a woman's heart and blood vessels by Leonardo da Vinci. The heart is in the middle of the drawing and opened to show the two main pumping chambers. The upper chamber is the left ventricle with the thicker muscular wall, which pumps blood into the aorta and its branches to supply the brain, arms, abdominal organs, and legs. The lower chamber is the right ventricle, which has a thinner muscular wall and receives blood from the body's veins and pumps blood to the lungs to pick up oxygen before heading to the left ventricle. *Source:* Science Photo Library, http://www.sciencephoto.com/

died from "failure of the artery which feeds the heart." He knew that healthy arteries had thin walls from a prior autopsy he'd performed on a child. But what did he mean by an artery that "feeds the heart?" Key to da Vinci's heart disease discovery was his prior discovery that the heart had special arteries to supply itself with oxygenated blood. His

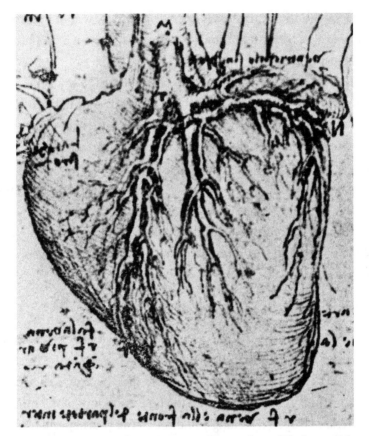

FIGURE 4.2   **Anatomic drawing of the surface of the heart with the coronary arteries by Leonardo da Vinci.** The main coronary artery comes out of the aorta (labeled *M* at the top of the drawing) and then branches across the surface of the heart to supply the muscle of the left ventricle to keep it pumping. Note the size of the coronary arteries is approximately one-tenth of an inch, and typically smaller in women than in men. *Source:* Science Photo Library, http://www.sciencephoto.com/

anatomic drawings and study of fluid flow convinced him that the small arteries he observed on the surface of the heart, what we now call the *coronary arteries,* were how the "heart feeds itself" (Figure 4.2). Thus, he discovered over 500 years ago that the main form of heart disease was not a problem of the heart muscle itself but abnormal thickening of the arteries that feed it, impairing blood flow. Little did he know that starting in the 1900s, this *coronary artery disease* would become the dominant cause of death causing heart attacks and sudden death in mid-life, not just in old age.

How did we go from beating heart muscle cells to thickened arteries to sudden death? Just like the body depends on the heart to beat every second of every day, the heart depends on these coronary arteries to supply the oxygenated blood it needs to keep beating. When the coronary arteries become diseased and narrowed, they can't supply enough blood for the heart to work. When the coronary arteries get plugged up suddenly, the starved heart muscle cells start to die—that's a *heart attack*. If it's a big heart attack, the heart stops pumping effectively, and we die suddenly. That's what happened to James Wu.

My Introduction to the Heart

Honestly, in my early cardiology career, neither I nor the cardiology community fully understood what was going on inside the thickened arteries that suddenly killed da Vinci's old man and my father-in-law. It took me time to fully understand the inner workings of the heart and blood vessels. Hopefully taking you through this journey will help your understanding as well.

It starts with the heart beating every second of every day. My introduction to heart disease was working as an engineering summer intern at the company that made the first pacemakers. A *pacemaker*, as the name implies, can take over the job of providing a regular electrical trigger to keep the heart beating. While it seems like a simple device—a battery with wires that contact the heart muscle—it was a revolutionary advance in medicine and remains a lifesaving technology.

Like the tech startups we know today, Earl Bakken, an engineer, founded Medtronic in a garage with his brother-in-law. This was in Minnesota, not California, and back in 1949, long before the development of the computer chips that gave Silicon Valley its name. They repaired hospital equipment and made devices for medical researchers. Bakken worked closely with a cardiac surgeon at the University of Minnesota who was pioneering open-heart surgery for children with congenital defects. Sometimes a successful heart repair would affect the ability of the heart muscle to pass its electrical signal from one part to the other. While a large external pacemaker had been built, children needed a smaller device that could keep them alive for a long time without depending on a wall outlet. Bakken found a design for a circuit that powered a metronome—another device that must beat regularly for a long time. Interestingly, the circuit was invented in MIT's Building 20, a "temporary" building constructed to help develop radar for World War II that later housed the Biomedical Engineering Center, where I did my senior thesis research.

Crazy as it may sound today, Bakken's first prototype went from garage to lab to patient in 24 hours. His small box had a nine-volt battery, wires to attach to the heart, and dials to adjust the rate and strength of the electrical stimulus. He drove it over to the animal lab at the university and it worked. Unbeknownst to him, the surgeon heard about it and needed it for a child whose heart was beating too slowly after surgery. The next day, Bakken went to the animal lab but found the box at the child's bedside, with the wires going into their chest to keep their heart beating—like a metronome. With the development of a strap to hold the box in place, this became the first "wearable" and let pacemaker patients become independent.

When I came to Medtronic's headquarters for the summer, they'd figured out how to miniaturize the box so it could be implanted under the skin with the wires going into the heart. Pacemakers had also become smarter in that the wires could also detect the electrical activity of the heart, producing what we call an *electrocardiogram* (ECG; electro=electrical, cardio=heart, gram=picture; you may also see it spelled EKG from the early German spelling). These smarter pacemakers would analyze the ECG to detect when the heart beat on its own and only trigger when it didn't. Pacemakers, however, weren't as smart about helping the heart beat faster when people were more active. Our resting heart rate is typically around 60 beats per minute (once every second), but it has to double or triple to pump more blood when we exercise. My summer project was about making pacemakers smarter. It turned out to be my introduction to ultrasound and the potential for imaging the heart, which later became a focus of my cardiology career.

Ultrasound involves sending out sound waves and listening for when some of them bounce back, like an echo, when they hit different parts of the body. The longer it takes for them to come back, the farther away something is. The project was to look at ways a pacemaker could go beyond keeping track of the ECG. If ultrasound could monitor how well the heart was working as a pump, it would tell the pacemaker if it needed to speed up to pump more blood with activity or slow down. This is what we now call a more personalized or "closed-loop" system— measuring and adjusting for the needs of the user. Because a pacemaker wire goes inside the right ventricle, could a small ultrasound device attached to that wire keep track of the ventricle's pumping and provide that information to the pacemaker? I wish I could say I was smart enough to have figured that out in a few months. Instead, experienced engineers at Medtronic figured out a simple and effective approach. The crystal material used for ultrasound can also pick up vibrations from movement, like the accelerometer crystals in phones and wearables that track movements and step counts. This small crystal was placed inside the pacemaker and could tell it to speed up the heartbeat when it detected more activity and slow down at rest. My contribution was not as an engineer but as a research subject. I wore a prototype on the outside of my chest and an ECG monitor for 24 hours, a setup that captured both the activity signal from the accelerometer and my heart rate while I biked to and from work, went for a run, and played tennis. When I returned the next summer, they showed me the poster they presented at a scientific meeting with a graph of the data— the new activity sensor tracked my heart rate almost perfectly! This became the Activitrax—the first "rate-responsive" pacemaker that helped patients be more active.

Starting My Imaging Career

Years later, when I became a cardiology fellow at Brigham & Women's Hospital in Boston, I thought I already knew how the heart worked. I studied beating frog hearts as an undergraduate. As a teaching assistant, one of my jobs was to pick up beef hearts from a nearby slaughterhouse—they were twice the size of a human heart and, thus, useful to teach students about the chambers and valves. I was appreciative in medical school of the people who donated their bodies so we could examine their hearts and learn their intricate details. On my clinical rotations, I learned how to read ECGs, listen to heart sounds, and appreciate the symptoms of chest pain and shortness of breath when patients came to the hospital.

Yet it became clear, early in my cardiology fellowship, that there was so much more to learn about the heart. In my second month, I was assigned to the echo lab. Echo is short for *echocardiogram*, a test that uses ultrasound to take pictures of the heart (pictures are formed from the echo of the sound waves bouncing back). Ultrasound imaging had become more sophisticated since my summer intern days at Medtronic. The ultrasound beam could sweep across the heart and process all the echoes quickly, so it could produce not just a still picture but a video of the heart structures as they moved. Most people have heard of this from ultrasounds of babies when they're still kicking in the womb. I still get goosebumps when I think of the first time a fetal ultrasound showed us Kelly's beating heart—all four chambers working together. It amazes me that you can watch the human heart beating, with the valves taking turns opening and closing, ensuring the body is getting its vital blood supply. From that moment on, the engineer in me was hooked.

The math and physics that went into this ultrasound machine allowed me to put a probe on someone's chest, see inside their heart, and determine if it was working well. I didn't get far with my ultrasound summer project at Medtronic, but now echo could easily see the pumping function of both the right and left ventricles, all from the outside (what we term *noninvasive imaging*). There would be so much to see—and learn—about the heart if I could master the echocardiogram.

My first echo research project taught me how the blood vessels can be just as important as the heart muscle in heart disease. Dr. Patricia Come was a cardiologist and echo specialist at the Brigham during my fellowship. She had graduated with honors from Harvard Medical School and became a faculty member at the Brigham. She was even rumored to be a character in the rite-of-passage book for medical trainees, *House of God*.[18] The Brigham pioneered using new blood-clot-busting drugs to treat cardiovascular disease under Dr. Eugene Braunwald. Dr. Come had started looking at echocardiograms in patients with blood clots in the *pulmonary arteries* that take blood from the right ventricle to the lungs. She noticed that right ventricle pumping decreased when a large clot blocked blood flow in the pulmonary arteries (what we call a *pulmonary embolism*). If patients underwent successful clot-busting drug treatment, the right ventricle could return to normal. One of the challenges of providing this lifesaving treatment was knowing whether a patient had a pulmonary embolism in the first place. Not surprisingly, it can cause chest pain and shortness of breath, but heart attacks are more common. Doctors don't always think of pulmonary embolism, delaying treatment. Serena Williams has been public about her history of pulmonary embolism and having to convince her doctors she was having another one after her daughter's birth (see FHDLC.info/SerenaInterview).[19] While Dr. Come had described many findings on echos that went with pulmonary embolism, she and Dr. Richard Lee, head of the Brigham echo lab, recommended that I analyze them in more detail. Because I still had some computer skills then, I could quantify how the right ventricle squeezed during a pulmonary embolism versus other conditions. We found that part of the right ventricle kept squeezing well while another part didn't—a distinct pattern that could distinguish a pulmonary embolism from other conditions.[20] Dr. Sam Goldhaber, who had overseen the clinical trials of the clot-busting drugs for pulmonary embolism, added this finding to his lectures and a review article in the *New England Journal of Medicine*, calling the echo finding "McConnell's sign."[21] This showed me the power of imaging. I'm appreciative of the opportunity given to me by the experienced cardiologists guiding me on that project.

Understanding Our Heart's Achilles Heel

We started with how the heart is a pump with muscle cells that beat on their own and pass their electrical signal to each other to beat in unison. We can see this with an ECG. When there are problems with the heartbeat, we can treat them with a pacemaker. Then we discussed how this pump connects to arteries that carry blood to other parts of the body. When blood flow gets blocked, as with pulmonary embolism, the heart can struggle, but it can recover if the blood clot is dissolved.

This leads us back to the main form of heart disease—coronary artery disease—which, as da Vinci discovered long ago, occurs when blood flow is blocked in the arteries that feed the heart itself. Without blood supply, the heart will struggle to keep beating and pumping, leading the heart—and life—to stop.

Heart cells, like every other cell, need a supply of oxygen and energy to keep working. Da Vinci's anatomic drawings showed that the coronary arteries emerge from the aorta and make a U-turn back to the heart. They extend along the surface, giving off small branches to supply the heart muscle. He wrote that the heart "is nourished by an artery and veins, as are other muscles." When you first think about this, it doesn't make sense. The heart is filled with blood, so why would it need special arteries for its blood supply? Da Vinci's dissections showed that the heart had these arteries like other parts of the body, so he came to this logical conclusion. The blood flowing inside the heart can only supply oxygen and nutrients to the inner layer of cells. The human heart has many cell layers—it needs to be a thick muscle to pump blood to the whole body, especially against gravity to supply the brain as we walk upright. Thus, coronary arteries go along the outside of the heart and send branches into the muscle so every cell gets its supply. This adaptation allows us to have bigger, thicker, and stronger hearts that beat continuously.

But this positive adaptation has become our biggest vulnerability—our Achilles heel. Any problem that develops in our small coronary arteries threatens the pump that keeps us alive. Da Vinci recognized the cruel irony in this vulnerability when he dissected the heart and vessels of the old man who died suddenly—the heart that supplied blood to the whole body couldn't feed itself because of disease in its own artery supply. We finally get to the source of the problem, and that's why the main medical term for heart disease is coronary artery disease. Our greatest killer doesn't start in the heart itself but as a growth inside a small vessel that we can't see or feel.

MRI and the Tenth of an Inch Problem

Having learned the power of ultrasound to see the heart from the outside and detect a blood clot in the pulmonary artery, I naturally wanted to see inside the heart arteries to detect coronary artery disease.

The standard technique, which remains the gold standard today, was for cardiologists to perform a *coronary angiogram* (angio=vessel, gram=picture) by inserting a tube (catheter) into an arm or leg artery, sliding it backward through the aorta to the heart, and squirting dye into the coronary arteries while taking x-rays. This lets us watch the dye flow through the arteries for any narrowing. It's a lifesaving technique during a heart attack because it can show the blockage and guide where to use a balloon catheter to open it and place a metal stent, restoring blood flow. Still, a coronary angiogram is not a simple procedure and not what you'd want to have as a screening test. While it's a low-risk procedure overall, some people experience complications or reactions to the dye. In my first month as a cardiology fellow, I saw several patients with severe coronary narrowing have their symptoms or blood pressure worsen from the stress of the procedure and be rushed to emergency cardiac surgery. So while this coronary angiogram makes sense to guide lifesaving interventions, it shouldn't be used as an early test for disease. There had to be a better way to see the coronary arteries without an invasive procedure.

This brings up what I call "the tenth of an inch problem." When teaching about the heart, I ask students how big they think the arteries are that supply the heart—not their length but the diameter of the inner *lumen* where blood flows. Many reply "an inch" or "half an inch," and all are surprised when I answer "one-tenth of an inch." This is only a bit thicker than the width of spaghetti or a toothpick. With that realization, they're much less surprised that it doesn't take much disease inside these arteries to cause big problems.

It's also not a surprise that this presented a major challenge to imaging the coronary arteries from the outside. Ultrasound can image larger vessels or those close to the surface of the body, but it can't reliably image the spaghetti-sized coronary arteries as they course along the surface of the heart deep within the chest.

Thankfully, I'd heard about another MIT-trained engineer and cardiologist, Warren Manning, who was working on this exact problem. He worked at Beth Israel Hospital, another Harvard teaching hospital next door to the Brigham. He became another key mentor for my clinical and research career. He was working with radiologists and engineers on using *magnetic resonance imaging* (MRI) to see the heart and coronary arteries.

You may be familiar with MRI if you've been checked for damage in your knees or a bulging disc in your back. I've had both! Like ultrasound, MRI can see internal structures without dye or x-rays. It uses a powerful magnet to detect the vibrations (resonance) of the water molecules in the body to form pictures. These molecules vibrate differently for different body parts, so MRI is great for seeing different structures inside the knee or back. Its earliest clinical application was seeing cancer because tumors looked different by MRI.

MRI of the heart has had an extra challenge—the heart moves. While echo can generate images in real time as the heart beats, MRI needed more time to add up all the small signals from the vibrating water molecules to make a clear picture. That's not an issue for the knee or back because those don't move on their own, but the heart must keep moving. It turns out that the ECG lets us "freeze" the heart motion to get a clear picture. Remember when we talked about pacemakers? They detect when the heart beats and can trigger a heartbeat if needed. A cardiac MRI does something similar. We place a few ECG electrodes on a patient's chest when they go into the scanner so it can keep track of when the heart beats. The heart's motion pauses briefly between beats. A cardiac MRI can use that still period to acquire its data over several heartbeats, "freezing" the heart motion. Voila—those small coronary arteries now show up in the image rather than being blurry due to motion.

Of course, I left one important thing out—something we don't think of regarding heart motion. The heart shares space inside the chest with the lungs, and the bottom of it sits on top of the diaphragm—the muscle that moves up and down to pull air into the lungs as we breathe. Tracking the ECG helped solve part of the problem, but we needed to keep patients' breathing from moving the heart up and down and causing blurry pictures. You may have guessed the easiest solution—stop breathing! Then the diaphragm would stay still so we could get sharp pictures. That's exactly what we did in the beginning—we combined the ECG with asking patients to hold their breath during the scan. That worked well enough to see the coronary arteries emerge from the aorta, as da Vinci had drawn 500 years before.

This technique enabled my first research project using cardiac MRI to see problems with the coronary arteries.[22] It turns out that almost one out of every hundred people are born with variations in how the coronary arteries emerge from the aorta. Perhaps if da Vinci had done a few more dissections, he'd have been the first to discover this too. The good news is that most of these "coronary anomalies" are benign, but a few can be lethal, and studies of cardiac arrest in young athletes show that coronary anomalies are a common cause.[23] Normally, the coronary artery that supplies the left side of the heart emerges from the left side of the aorta. The most dangerous abnormalities are when the coronary artery comes off the "wrong" side—the left coronary artery comes off the right side or vice versa. Why is that a problem? Two issues are often present—to cross back to the other side of the heart, the artery must make a sharp turn and go between the aorta and the pulmonary artery. When a garden hose is bent too much, flow can decrease. Also, a small coronary artery between the larger aorta and pulmonary artery can get squeezed, particularly when these big arteries are pulsing more vigorously during exercise. In our study, we used MRI to get clear images of many types of coronary anomalies, relying on the ECG and breath-holding techniques. Cardiac MRI is now a standard noninvasive way to look for this important form of congenital heart disease.[24]

To find coronary artery disease, however, we wanted to see not just the path of the artery, but inside it to detect whether it was narrowed due to plaque buildup. Given that the artery is one-tenth of an inch, to measure any narrowing, we'd need to see even more detail. For MRI, that required scanning longer for more data—longer than people can hold their breath. The second trick we used to freeze heart motion for longer scans was to track our breathing like we used ECG to track our heartbeat. Engineers had figured out how to use part of the time that MRI was scanning the heart to quickly scan the diaphragm. This gives a real-time signal of the diaphragm position, which can guide when and where to take the heart artery pictures. Just like we used the ECG to take pictures when the heart was between beats, we could make sure the patient was between breaths. To make it more accurate, if someone's diaphragm doesn't return to the exact level, the software could adjust where to take the MRI picture.[25] This is like how smartphone cameras correct for hand movements when we take selfies, adjusting the camera so the picture stays sharp. This allowed patients to breathe normally and us to image longer for detailed pictures of the coronary arteries.

This cardiovascular MRI technology became the initial focus of my research and clinical career. The quest to see inside the heart arteries and the plaques growing there—especially whether they're malignant—would take me well beyond MRI. More to come.

There you have it—the heart disease that is, in many ways, worse than cancer, lives and grows inside the tiny coronary arteries that supply our hearts. Like many cardiologists, detecting this growth, knowing when it's malignant, and helping to prevent and reverse its consequences became the basis for my career. Knowing where heart disease starts is just the beginning. Being able to do something about it, for yourself and your loved ones, is what's important. Applying the lessons of cancer is how I'll help you do that.

CHAPTER 5

How Can "Tumors" Cause Heart Attacks?

"Tumors" in the Heart

Hopefully you now understand that the main form of heart disease doesn't start in the heart muscle itself but in the small coronary arteries—the "plumbing" that supplies the heart. That's where the abnormal tissue growth—or tumor—begins. So, are there really tumors growing in the heart? In what should have been considered a "spoiler alert," several cardiology and pathology colleagues asked this question over 20 years ago and published an article describing the many ways that coronary plaque could be considered "a cancer of the blood vessels."[26] Unfortunately, we're still overdue to share that knowledge with our patients. I want to have the same straight talk with you that I have with my Stanford Preventive Cardiology Clinic patients. I want to help you see heart disease in this new light that the latest science is showing us.

Unfortunately, we've had to rediscover this science multiple times over the history of medicine. We discussed earlier that the first indication was from da Vinci comparing the arteries of an old man who died suddenly to those of a young child and finding artery "thickening." While this doesn't sound like cancer, the first medical term for this disease—*atheroma*—certainly does. It's from the Greek words for tumor (-oma) and gruel (athero-) because they saw that the artery wall had a tumor filled with fatty gruel. This term may sound familiar because

Hippocrates first described cancerous tumors with a similar word: *carcinoma*, meaning a "crab-shaped" tumor of a skin cancer he saw. In the late 1800s, Rudolf Virchow, the father of modern pathology, studied these atheromas under the microscope and indeed found that these growths had many features similar to carcinoma (Figure 5.1).

Virchow's discoveries and efforts to teach about them are a great lesson. He was an expert at studying disease under the microscope and found things that didn't match the classic teachings derived from the pre-microscope days of Hippocrates a thousand years before. Virchow

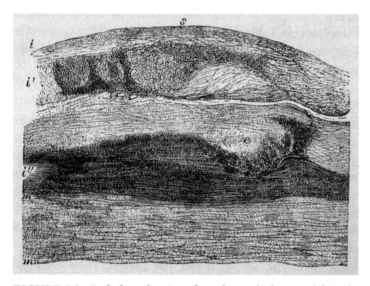

FIGURE 5.1   Pathology drawing of an advanced atheroma (plaque) within the wall of an artery by Rudolph Virchow. A healthy artery wall would primarily just have the layer of muscle, labeled *m* at the bottom of the drawing. Instead, there are multiple complex layers (*i'* and *i"*) that have developed and pushed the surface (*s*) of the wall up into the lumen of the artery where the blood flows. Virchow described very well the complex growth of these "malignant" plaques, with areas of proliferation (*i'*), areas of fatty degeneration (*i"*), and areas transitioning from proliferation to degeneration (*e*). *Source*: Virchow R. Lecture XVI—Atheromatous affection of arteries. In *Cellular Pathology as Based Upon Physiological and Pathological Histology* [. . .]. Robert M. De Witt; 1858

could see what was happening at the cellular level, writing that "the science of pathology" is based on "the cellular nature of all vital processes."
He wanted to update practitioners on this new science because he saw
teachings as being "transmitted from the mythic days of antiquity" with
a "mechanical and chemical bias." He decided he needed to give a series
of lectures to explain his discoveries under the microscope and show
that disease is caused by cells going awry. Thankfully for us, he worked
with a colleague to compile all these lectures into a book, complete with
drawings, for posterity and so his modern science of the time could be
distributed more widely.[27] He wanted to "fulfill the duties both of an
observer and of an instructor." He highlighted a regular challenge in
medicine, even in today's "information age"—the time demands of providing patient care make it hard to stay up to date on the latest science.
He saw that practitioners "consume their best energies," making it "less
and less possible . . . to understand the more recent medical works."

What did Virchow see and teach about atheroma and coronary
artery disease in the 1850s? His first comment, fittingly, is that this is a
topic where "confusion . . . has perhaps been the greatest." He laid out
the processes of atheroma development that match our current understanding. Under the microscope, he saw fat deposits ("fatty metamor-
phosis") in the vessel wall and described "inflammation of the inner
arterial wall as the starting point" of atheroma. He noted that this tumor could progress with degeneration of the wall and spread "without
any well-defined limits," and "the further this degeneration advances,"
the more it can become "like pus when an abscess is cut into." Importantly, he saw active, growing cells as key to this process. "The cellular
elements of the wall increase in size . . . division occurs in the cells . . .
an active process, which really produces new tissues, and then hurries
on to destruction." He even presages the "tip of the iceberg" concept
we'll discuss—"in the extreme stage," an atheroma "deep beneath the . . .
surface . . . bursts . . . leading to just as destructive results as we see in
the course of other violent inflammatory processes."

What Virchow described so well almost 200 years ago was how we have complex, growing tumors in our vessels with fatty infiltration, inflammation, and ultimate destruction of the vessel wall with "violent" consequences—what we now call *plaque rupture*. This complex, active biology is a far cry from the simpler notion I first learned of a slow-growing plumbing or mechanical problem.

So how was it that most physicians, when I was learning medicine, still viewed coronary disease as a gradual buildup of plaque inside the vessel rather than a complex growing tumor that could burst violently? Like many areas of progress in human knowledge, there were competing views. Often, the newer views take much longer to prevail. As Virchow indicated in the introduction to his lectures on this new *cellular pathology*—that cell abnormalities were the basis of disease—he was trying to overturn the older views "from antiquity." Shockingly, the view of health and disease in Virchow's day was still based on theories that started with Hippocrates 2,000 years earlier—that they were related to the balance of humors—blood, bile, and phlegm. Indeed, there was a competing view of atherosclerosis that it was due to blood abnormalities. Another famous pathologist—Carl von Rokitansky—theorized that components of the blood caused the "encrustation" of the vessel wall he saw. We'll discuss in more detail the contribution of blood clots to heart attacks, but the origin of the disease is very much the growing atheroma tumor Virchow described.

Hippocrates was also famous for the Hippocratic Oath physicians take in their training, a key part of which is simplified to "do no harm." Physicians are taught to be cautious in following new science or treatment to minimize the risk of harm, but this can make it easy to continue current practice. That's part of why Virchow went around giving his lectures. He realized that busy physicians don't have time to learn the most modern science. I wish, in my training, we'd read his book, but I'm glad we've rediscovered his work. Now it's our turn to convey this modern science to more patients and providers.

Narrowed Pipes Are Not the Full Story

When I graduated medical school, the worlds of heart disease and cancer couldn't seem further apart, except they competed to kill the most people in the United States. Heart disease specialists like cardiologists and cardiac surgeons and companies like Medtronic and General Electric had developed new health technologies with which we could take pictures of narrowed arteries and use bypass surgery or balloon catheters to improve blood flow to the heart. We thought we had this cured.

Still, people like my father-in-law were having heart attacks, often without warning. We'd forgotten what pathologists like Virchow had shown us. We were approaching heart disease like engineers or plumbers, thinking that plaque would slowly clog the heart arteries (the pipes). Then the decreased blood flow would cause warning symptoms of chest pain (*angina*), which we could "fix" by opening the narrowings (what we call *coronary angioplasty*) or routing blood around them with new pipes (what we call *coronary artery bypass* surgery).

That sounds simple to understand and not particularly scary. So why were we seeing patients come into the ER with heart attacks who never had symptoms of clogged arteries or patients with a normal "stress test" die of a heart attack the next day? Thankfully, researchers started taking a careful look—again.

Silent Growth, like Cancer

One fundamental reason our approach wasn't working is that plaques can grow for a long time without causing symptoms. Thus, heart disease can be "silent" until it's too late. Most cancers also grow silently, as with my grandfather and my sister, who only developed symptoms after her cancer spread toward her liver.

Why don't these plaques cause symptoms until late? Didn't we say that these coronary arteries are only one-tenth of an inch, so it shouldn't take much plaque to cause a narrowing? Well, there are several parts to the answer.

The first is that, like most everything about the human body, we have methods to adapt. Plaques are sneaky—they can grow without causing narrowing. How can that happen and how did we learn that? Pathologists started comparing the amount of plaque they saw with the degree of narrowing in the artery. They saw many areas along the artery with a large plaque, but the inner channel (*lumen*) where blood flows wasn't narrowed. Our arteries were adapting! As plaques grew, the artery got larger so the lumen could stay big enough for unimpeded blood flow. Detailed measurements from autopsies showed that the heart arteries enlarge when plaques grow, preserving blood flow.[28] Only when a plaque gets very big does the artery fail to compensate. Then the additional growth narrows the lumen.

The second part of the answer is another way our arteries compensate. You might think that once the lumen starts to narrow, we get symptoms, but that occurs only when it's advanced. The main coronary arteries don't actually control blood flow to the heart as much as the millions of artery branches and capillaries that follow. When narrowing causes increased resistance to blood flow, we dilate the vessels downstream to keep flow normal. When researchers quantified the narrowing required to cause a decrease in flow, it was close to 90%! That was when they tested at rest, but it meant that our heart circulation could compensate a lot to keep blood flowing. Maybe you've heard about the classic symptom of heart disease—chest pain when walking fast, exercising, or shoveling snow. What's that about? The heart muscle needs up to five times as much blood flow when we exercise. That's why I ask patients whether they have symptoms when they walk up stairs or a hill. That's also why we conduct stress tests. When you increase the demand on the heart, the supply must increase. A more modest narrowing can make the supply inadequate for the demand. Again, researchers have looked at this and it still takes more than 50% narrowing to impact blood flow and cause symptoms with exercise.

"Malignant" Plaques

So far, it sounds good that our heart arteries are resilient. They can expand to accommodate plaque growth and compensate to provide good flow when partially narrowed. The downside to these adaptive mechanisms, which is where the cancer aspect comes in most clearly, is that plaques can grow silently from small to large (and, as we'll describe, from benign to malignant) without warning.

The third part of the answer is the main problem in the end. When a plaque becomes malignant, it can cause a heart attack without much narrowing. The first two parts explained why the heart can adapt to plaques growing over time, delaying the severe narrowing that causes warning signs and symptoms. As they grow silently, their biology can become more complex and deadly. Recall Virchow's description of plaque inflammation like pus that can burst. We know that plaque buildup starts early—pathologists analyzing the heart arteries of young soldiers killed in battle showed that even these 20-year-olds had early atheroma forming. But pathologists found very different plaques when they studied patients who died from heart attacks, with complex biology more like cancer, namely areas of inflammation and angiogenesis (i.e., new blood vessel growth, which we'll explain later). These complex biological features, we've learned, make plaques vulnerable to causing a heart attack. They no longer simply grow slowly. I call them malignant plaques because they're biologically active and don't remain contained or benign. Indeed, they result in cracks, tears, or rupture of the plaque surface, exposing the inside of the plaque to the blood flowing in the coronary lumen. The blood tries to do its job of forming a clot where there's a crack or rupture, but a clot inside the artery can completely block flow.

That's the cascade of events of a heart attack—a plaque hiding deep inside the vessel wall, not causing significant narrowing, can rupture and trigger a blood clot that blocks blood flow and kills the heart muscle cells downstream. It's this aspect that's worse than cancer—our coronary arteries can go from good blood flow to completely blocked in minutes. That's how my father-in-law could get on a van feeling fine and not get off. He had the ultimate form of malignant tumor in his heart arteries.

Science has continued to show us the similarities between heart disease and cancer. The cell growth, inflammation, and angiogenesis are common features of both malignant plaques and cancer. Peter Libby, one of my mentors at the Brigham, in reviewing the current view that inflammation is key to plaque development, acknowledges that Virchow had it right almost 200 years ago and we've had it wrong.[29] "Over the last quarter century, the concept that inflammation plays a primordial role in atherogenesis has gained ascendancy. Yet, as with many innovations in science and medicine, the roots of this seemingly modern concept stretch far back in time." To truly see heart disease and understand its risk, we needed to see more than the pipes. We needed to see the plaques themselves and understand when they posed a risk—were they malignant or benign? Contrary to what I first learned, the biology of heart disease was much more important than the plumbing.

Imaging under the "Tip of the Iceberg"

One of the big paradigm shifts away from the conventional "plumbing" view of heart disease was the discovery that when we saw plaques narrowing the artery on an angiogram, we were only seeing the "tip of the iceberg." Thus, our gold-standard test for heart disease wasn't really seeing the plaques themselves. As discussed above, plaques can grow and evolve for some time—"hiding" in the artery wall. Pathologists had been showing us that there could be big plaques inside the wall, and that in people who died of a heart attack, there was evidence that they had burst, blocking blood flow in the artery. But pathologists couldn't tell us what the plaque that caused the heart attack had looked like the year before. That's where imaging came in. An angiogram is often done during or after a heart attack to see where the blockage is so further treatment can be planned. Some patients who had an angiogram during their heart attack also had one to evaluate chest pain months or years before the heart attack.[30] This let cardiology researchers compare the new angiogram showing the location of the blockage causing the heart attack to the prior angiogram. It turned out that most of the new heart attacks were caused by plaques that hadn't caused severe narrowing before. Indeed, over two-thirds were caused by plaques with less than 50% narrowing. Similarly, the branch of the coronary artery with the most severe narrowing was typically not where the heart attack occurred. There was also no relationship between the severity of narrowing and how soon a heart attack would occur. This simple study of only 29 patients completely upended our view of coronary artery disease at the time. We had thought plaques became progressively more severe, leading to heart attacks. We expected the study to show that the severe narrowings on the first angiogram would be the ones that caused the blockage and heart attack on the second angiogram and that the more severe the narrowing, the sooner a heart attack would occur. The opposite was found, and the study's conclusion summarized it well—the "severity of coronary stenosis may be inadequate to accurately predict the time or location of a subsequent coronary occlusion." The severe narrowings we focused on didn't predict when or where a heart attack would occur! If anything, the more moderate narrowings were the main culprits. How could this be? This didn't make sense to the engineer in me. It meant that the biology of these plaques must be more complex than we appreciated. It did help explain the conundrum of how patients without chest pain could still have heart attacks. It even explained how a patient could have a normal stress test one day, meaning no severe narrowing, and a heart attack the next, something even scarier than cancer!

Before we get to the complex biology, this study also showed us that the angiogram was not the best way to see how much plaque is in the arteries. An angiogram is not a picture of the plaque. It's a picture from the dye we inject, so it shows the blood flowing in the lumen. We learned earlier that the artery expands as plaques grow, an adaptation that keeps the lumen the same size for good blood flow. So, like with an iceberg seen from above the surface of the ocean, the narrowing on the angiogram is just the tip of the plaque and doesn't tell us how much plaque has grown in the wall below.

But how could we know that the angiogram was only seeing the tip of the iceberg? Pathologists had been seeing that plaques could grow quite large within the artery wall before they started to narrow the "pipe" where the blood flowed. There was the famous study in the *New England Journal of Medicine* that analyzed the plaques from 136 hearts at autopsy. [28] Their conclusion was prescient—"The preservation of a nearly normal lumen cross-sectional area despite the presence of a large plaque should be taken into account in evaluating atherosclerotic disease [plaque] with use of coronary angiography." They were cluing us into the idea that the angiogram is not the best test for plaque buildup!

Could there be a better imaging test to see the plaque building up inside the wall—the whole iceberg? There are now several, but the first was ultrasound. If you remember, I described how the echocardiogram uses ultrasound to bounce sound waves off tissue to look at the heart muscle and valves. But I also said the heart arteries were too small for the echocardiogram to work well enough to see coronary plaque buildup. What gives? Well, I was talking about ultrasound from outside the body. What if you could do ultrasound from *inside* the heart arteries? Up close, the ultrasound probe can use higher frequency sound waves to see smaller structures, like plaque.

But how do you get ultrasound inside a heart artery? Paul Yock, a longtime Stanford colleague and friend, was drawn to imaging the heart during cardiology fellowship, like me. He similarly benefited from the mentorship of Stanford echo pioneer Richard Popp. But Dr. Yock also became interested in *interventional cardiology*—using catheters not just for angiograms but for interventions using balloons and, later, stents to open coronary blockages. He figured out how to combine his two areas of expertise and put a small ultrasound probe at the end of a catheter to take pictures of plaque up close.[31] This *intravascular ultrasound* could image the coronary artery wall, not just the lumen, and see—before a heart attack occurred—that large plaques were hiding without severely narrowing the lumen. In a classic Silicon Valley story, he obtained a patent, founded a company, and launched his career as an inventor, entrepreneur, and cardiologist. With my MIT friend Josh Makower, he cofounded the Stanford Biodesign program that has taught medical innovation to hundreds of young doctors, engineers, and entrepreneurs over the last 20 years (see FHDLC.info/Biodesign)![32]

This inspired us to focus our MRI research on imaging the vessel wall in addition to the lumen. We showed that we could now see large plaques within the wall noninvasively—without inserting a catheter. Earlier, we discussed my initial use of MRI to perform a coronary angiogram noninvasively to detect narrowing. That used a technique called *bright-blood* MRI, in which flowing blood looks bright on the image, like an angiogram. There was also a *black-blood* technique that instead makes flowing blood look dark and the wall look bright. Others had shown that this technique makes it easier to see plaque in the walls of larger vessels, so we adapted it to see plaque buildup in coronary arteries. We saw what intravascular ultrasound was seeing—the angiogram could look OK, but in some people, plaque was already there. We could see the "iceberg" before the artery narrowed. [33,34]

Because MRI was noninvasive, we could monitor plaques over time. We knew high cholesterol causes plaques to grow, but we understood less how much they could improve with a low cholesterol diet. In my first study combining technology and prevention, we used MRI to test high and low cholesterol diets over time. We used animals to avoid causing high cholesterol and plaque buildup in humans. As expected, MRI showed plaque buildup over time during the high cholesterol diet, but part way through the study, we put some animals back on their normal, low cholesterol diets. While MRI showed plaques in the high cholesterol group continued to grow, we saw reversal of plaque growth in the low cholesterol group—more on that to come.[35]

Putting this all together, we realized that heart disease can develop silently, with plaques growing without warning of an imminent heart attack, and imaging technologies were starting to detect this noninvasively.[36] But we also knew that plaque buildup was common and started early. What we still needed to know was which patients, or even which plaques, were at high risk of causing a heart attack. Thus emerged the concept of "vulnerable" versus "stable" plaques. I began to describe this to my patients in cancer terms—"malignant" versus "benign." We discussed how most plaques that build up inside the artery wall don't cause narrowing, so flow is preserved. If they stayed like that, heart disease would be quite benign. Even if plaques grew slowly, causing gradual narrowing, that would still be relatively benign because we have procedures—stents, bypass surgery—to treat this. It's the heart attacks that are the truly malignant part of heart disease, as they can happen unexpectedly and destroy heart muscle and cause the heart to stop. Like cancer, we need to understand and detect the biology of heart disease if we are to convert it from malignant to benign. That could have helped prevent the malignant heart "tumor" that killed my father-in-law.

CHAPTER 6

Beyond "Tumors" in the Heart

We've focused on the main killer in heart disease—the plaque "tumors" growing in the heart arteries that cause heart attacks and sudden death. Unfortunately, the same risk factors can promote plaque growth in other arteries and contribute to other forms of heart and vessel (cardiovascular) disease. While there are entire books on these, it's helpful to be aware of them. Importantly, many of the prevention and treatment approaches we'll discuss below can help. Feel free to skip this chapter to keep learning how to fight heart disease like cancer and turn it benign. However, I didn't want to delay the important discussion of women's heart disease and the many other forms of cardiovascular disease that can be helped.

Women Get Heart Disease Too, in More Ways Than One

Women also die of heart disease at high rates and are prone to the same plaque tumors as men but women often have other forms of disease in their coronary arteries. When I discussed this book with my now grown-up daughters, Mia brought up how her risk for heart disease doesn't come up when she sees her doctor:

As a woman, one of the earliest, and only, illnesses I have feared is breast cancer. The moment that my female body began to develop, my pediatrician added an additional routine to my check ups—checking my breasts for abnormal lumps. She informed me of the high risk of breast cancer, asked about my family's history of breast cancer, and reminded me to routinely perform self-check ups on my breasts to check for cancerous lumps. Once I reached the age of needing a gynecologist, I began to receive routine Pap smears once a year to check for cervical cancer. And yet again, when I turn 40, I will have doctors inform me to start going in for my yearly mammogram as they highlight the likelihood of breast cancer and remind me to stay alert for unusual changes in my breasts. Don't get me wrong, it is so important to be aware of these cancers and I'm so appreciative of my doctors for educating me on how to detect early signs of breast cancer. However, what was left out of all of these visits and conversations was any mention of a far more deadly and widespread threat—heart disease. A disease that "disables and kills more women than all cancers combined" (from Women are Not Small Men*[37]). Why is it that I, to this day, have never been informed about the likelihood of heart disease in my doctor's office? Never asked if my parents or grandparents have had heart ailments? Never educated on what symptoms of heart disease could look like? Never taught that symptoms of heart disease look different in men and women? Since I was old enough to understand breast cancer, I have feared that I or other women in my life would get the unlucky news of being the one in the eight women who get diagnosed. What I have neither feared nor known is the fact that the chances of a woman dying from heart disease are one in three. The chances of dying from breast cancer are one in thirty. Not only is heart disease a worse threat to women than breast cancer, but it actually is, on average, more deadly in women than in men—with more severe heart attacks, lower survival in the first year after a heart attack, and higher chances of getting a second heart attack. These are all statistics that I would be completely unaware of if I were not in the uncommon position of having a cardiologist as a father (which for a long time I resented because it meant a lot less ice cream and French fries). If my medical treatment as a woman reflected the relative risk of breast*

*cancer versus heart disease, I would've been hearing about heart dis-
ease just as early if not earlier on than I learned about breast cancer.*

Mia captured how we approach cancer more seriously than heart disease from education to early screening, especially in women. Heart
disease is viewed as less of a concern—by women themselves and their
physicians. This means prevention, screening, and treatment occur less
than in men, and outcomes are often worse. The AHA's Go Red for
Women campaign aims to bust the myths people have about heart disease in women (see FHDLC.info/GoRed).[38]

In medical school, we learned that estrogen protected women from
heart disease and that we should make sure they received it after menopause. This went with our historical understanding that women typically get heart disease later than men, and early menopause increases
risk for early disease. Plus, at the time, the clinical data were compelling, especially after publication of a 10-year study of almost 50,000
nurses. The nurses who opted to take estrogen had almost a 50% lower
risk of heart disease. But this was not a randomized trial where participants were randomly assigned estrogen or a placebo (fake pill). That's
the best way to know whether prescribing estrogen would help. When
a large, randomized trial in a broader population came out a few years
later, the results were the opposite. Women randomized to receive
estrogen had more heart attacks and other diseases involving blood
clots. Now I make sure my patients, particularly those with existing
heart disease, don't take hormone replacement therapy longer than
needed to manage their menopausal symptoms.

So, what is the current science on heart disease in women? Statistics are telling us, as Mia noted, that one in three women in the United
States will die of heart disease, yet less than half know it's their top health
risk! And while women may have some delay in having the typical heart
attack due to bursting plaques, they can develop other forms of disease
in their heart arteries. Maybe the data on women being "protected"
longer from heart disease exists, in part, because we physicians were

not looking carefully enough. We were looking for the typical male form of disease in women.

I learned this firsthand years ago when a middle-aged patient said she was having mild shortness of breath when walking briskly. She didn't have the typical angina (chest pain), but she was overweight with high blood pressure and diabetes. She thought it may be from being out of shape and needing more exercise, but it sounded more concerning than that. We did a stress test that didn't show evidence of a severe coronary blockage; however, stress tests aren't perfect, so we did an angiogram. This didn't show any typical plaques causing blockages, but she did have narrower vessels overall. She had a form of more diffuse disease in her coronary arteries rather than large plaques. We now recognize that this form of heart disease occurs more often in women. The coronary arteries can have diffusely thickened walls down to the smallest branches, which we call *microvascular disease*. This can also be associated with the arteries not dilating well when needed. We call this *endothelial dysfunction*, because the endothelium is the inner lining of the arteries that normally signals the arteries when to dilate. Both microvascular disease and endothelial dysfunction limit the ability of the heart arteries to increase blood flow during stress or exercise. My patient's shortness of breath and fatigue, which can be more common than angina in women, were most certainly due to this. Fortunately, when we lowered the high blood pressure, glucose, and lipids contributing to her condition by increasing physical activity and adjusting her medications, her symptoms resolved.

Importantly, there are now women's heart disease centers that focus on understanding sex differences in heart disease. This includes awareness of different symptoms and novel ways to evaluate and treat these additional types of coronary artery disease. Also, the AHA's Go Red for Women initiative includes educational campaigns to raise women's awareness of their risk and support more research to improve prevention, diagnosis, and treatment of heart disease in women. As Mia highlighted, this should be top of mind—like cancer—for women, not just men.

Extra Heart Muscle in the Wrong Place

We've discussed at length how heart disease is a problem of the coronary arteries rather than the heart muscle. There's a twist to this story, however, where extra heart muscle can cause a problem with our coronary blood supply. In humans, the coronary arteries travel along the heart's surface, as in Leonardo da Vinci's drawings. Small branches come off the surface arteries and go into the heart muscle. Some people, however, are born with a variation in this anatomy. This is not the coronary anomaly where the artery originates in the wrong place—the topic of my first MRI research paper. This is a more subtle variation where the artery dips down into the muscle for a short segment and then back to the surface. It becomes a "tunnel" under a "bridge" of heart muscle. The challenge is that this *myocardial bridge* squeezes with each heartbeat, like the rest of the heart muscle. This means that the artery under the bridge gets squeezed, limiting blood flow. The good news is that most of the blood flow through the coronary artery happens between heartbeats, while the heart muscle is relaxed. But when we exercise, the heart squeezes harder and faster, so the coronary artery gets more compressed and there's less time between heartbeats for blood to flow. In cardiology fellowship, we were taught that a myocardial bridge was a rare cause of heart disease—an interesting variant we might see on a board exam or in a journal report of an unusually severe case. But this variant turns out to be quite common.

One of my colleagues at Stanford has done a lot to improve our understanding of how a myocardial bridge is more of an issue than we thought. Dr. Ingela Schnittger was born in Sweden and came to the United States to train with Dr. Richard Popp, mentioned earlier as a mentor and one of the inventors of echocardiography and founder of the Stanford echo lab. I first met Dr. Schnittger when she was a young faculty member and I was a Stanford medical student. I remember her stories of reading early echo studies with Dr. Popp when it was all on paper, before they developed two-dimensional (2D) echo pictures or the 2D and 3D videos we see now. She had taught her husband, an anesthesiologist, about echo so he could help monitor the heart's status during an operation. Dr. Schnittger went on to become director of the Stanford Echo Lab, which I joined when I returned as an assistant professor.

Her myocardial bridge research started when she was investigating a complicated clinical case. Like my experienced colleagues at the Brigham who first noticed a change in how the heart squeezed in pulmonary embolism, Dr. Schnittger noted an unusual heart squeezing pattern during a stress echo. Usually, an echo stress test involves taking pictures of the heart beating before and after walking on a treadmill. A normal heart squeezes more vigorously after exercise, while a heart with a severe coronary artery narrowing (like from advanced plaque buildup) will stop squeezing in the region supplied by the narrowed coronary artery. What Dr. Schnittger noted in this case was that part of the heart didn't squeeze right but only during a brief part of the heartbeat. A typical blockage from plaque buildup causes the heart to squeeze poorly throughout the heartbeat. She wondered what could cause this problem for only part of the heartbeat. A myocardial bridge only compresses the artery when the heart squeezes but not when it relaxes between beats. Could this be the cause of what she was seeing? Figuring this out became a team effort. Many of us reviewed a series of patient cases—matching this brief squeezing problem during a stress test seen on echo (what I call the "Schnittger sign") with detailed analysis of the anatomy and flow changes in coronary arteries with myocardial bridges.[39] While this started as an interesting echo finding, through Dr. Schnittger's dedicated effort to translate this research into better care, she founded the Stanford Myocardial Bridge Center and helped pioneer better techniques to evaluate and treat bridges. Many patients came to see her with chest pain but no conventional blockages on their angiograms.

They'd been told there was nothing wrong with their hearts, even when they could no longer walk or do minimal exercise without having to stop from chest pain. She not only helped diagnose their myocardial bridges but helped them get curative treatment. Putting a metal stent in the coronary artery—as we do for severe coronary blockages—doesn't work for myocardial bridges. A stent is not designed to hold up to the constant squeezing and can fracture. Coronary bypass surgery doesn't always work because it doesn't help the blood flow where the myocardial bridge is. The most effective procedure is, perhaps, the most obvious— free the coronary artery segment from the heart muscle bridge so it doesn't get squeezed at all. This "unbridging" is called *unroofing* surgery and can be done safely with a small chest incision and without stopping the heart—amazing.

Another important twist to myocardial bridges—they can cause plaques! The squeezing with each heartbeat increases the blood's velocity in the coronary artery—just like when you put your thumb at the end of a garden hose to make the water jet out. This speeding up and slowing down of the blood along the coronary wall makes it prone to plaque formation. While the main lesson is that there are forms of coronary artery disease caused by anatomic variations that can impair flow and cause symptoms, myocardial bridges can also be a growth factor for coronary plaques.

Preventing Strokes ("Brain Attacks")

"Is it normal to get sent home from the emergency room with a stroke?" I'll always remember those words from my mother-in-law, Lily, when I took her call in an elevator at work at Brigham and Women's Hospital in Boston. Though I was still doing my cardiology fellowship, I knew enough to respond with "no." I explained that they usually keep you in the hospital to figure out the cause of the stroke and use intravenous blood thinners to dissolve any clot that contributed to it. She was calling about her brother, and I'll go into the rest of that story next.

Unfortunately, Lily had a small stroke herself a few years later. She was on a work trip with my father-in-law, James, and they didn't go to an emergency room or call me. Luckily, her symptoms resolved on their own, and she didn't tell anyone until she returned home.

Why are we talking about strokes? Throughout the book, I talk about preventing heart disease, but I noted that the most common issue starts in blood vessels. So, medically, we use the term *cardiovascular disease* (cardio=heart, vascular=vessels). It may seem confusing that we include strokes within that broader definition. That's because strokes typically come from our heart or blood vessels. The American Heart Association combined with the American Stroke Association several years ago because of their shared goals to promote cardiovascular and brain health and prevent both heart disease and stroke.

What is a *stroke*? It's like a heart attack, but the cells that die are in the brain, typically due to blocked blood flow. That's why a stroke can be considered a "brain attack." While stroke symptoms are very different from a heart attack, there should be the same urgency to get treatment—to save brain cells. The American Stroke Association and other groups have developed an acronym—FAST—to help people recognize stroke symptoms and take quick action. F is for face drooping, A is for arm weakness, S is for speech difficulty, and T is for time—time to call 911 (see FHDLC.info/FAST)![40] As with heart attacks, the main treatment for strokes has been to use strong blood thinners, clot-busting drugs, and/or catheters to remove clots in the brain arteries and restore blood flow. Strokes are a common form of cardiovascular disease and share many risk factors with heart attacks. In some parts of the world, strokes are more common than heart attacks. They can also be very debilitating, so prevention and rapid treatment can have a large impact on quality of life.

When Lily eventually let me know about her stroke symptoms, understanding more about why she had a stroke was essential to preventing another. She was only 60, and women having heart attacks or strokes before 65 is considered premature and means that her first-degree relatives, including my wife, are at higher risk. Lily Wu had attended the same top university in Taiwan as my father-in-law, James. She paused her graduate school studies to help raise her kids, but later completed her PhD and became a research scientist and faculty member at the University of Utah with James. Ironically, her expertise was in measuring the different forms of cholesterol and their risk for heart disease. The large Mormon population in Utah was particularly conducive to this research, especially the role of genetics, because they had large families and kept detailed records of their family trees. Researchers could study families with premature heart disease and high cholesterol, called *familial hypercholesterolemia* (FH), and find out how genes impacted cholesterol levels and contributed to this serious condition.

She did not have FH, but when we brought her to Stanford to get checked more thoroughly, she had the same plaque problem I've been describing. In her case, she had plaques in the vessels that supply the brain. These plaques were larger and visible on ultrasound. Her malignant plaque had likely burst, and the resulting clot had gone to her brain. Her brain attack was relatively mild, and she was able to get on the right therapy to reverse the risk factors making her plaques grow and burst, thankfully preventing another stroke.

While the plaques we've been discussing are scary in that they can cause heart attacks *and* strokes, the heart-healthy activities and risk factor control we'll discuss in later chapters can promote brain health and prevent strokes.[41] They can prevent a first stroke or, like my mother-in-law, prevent another potentially more disabling or lethal stroke.

Quivering Heart

"Is it normal to get sent home from the emergency room with a stroke?" I promised I'd tell you what happened to Lily's brother. He'd developed numbness in one arm and slurred speech (the A and S parts of FAST) and went to the emergency room. Thankfully, his symptoms had started to improve when he got there. Not so thankfully, the emergency room staff weren't convinced that his speech was still slurred, despite what his wife said, likely because English was his third language. Like my wife's parents, he was born in China. He had come to the United States after a stint working in Germany. When I spoke with him, he was already at home. He felt mostly better but had no idea why he had the stroke symptoms. I asked him about the tests they did. He said they did an ECG, which was abnormal, but they compared it to a prior ECG and let him go home because there was no change.

I asked him about this prior ECG. He recalled that he'd done it for a work physical exam, and they told him to get it checked out. He hadn't gotten around to doing that yet, but he had a copy at home. I asked him to get it so we could talk through it over the phone. This was before smartphones, where one could just take a picture of the ECG and send it via text message. An ECG waveform, like you've probably seen on TV (and on the cover of this book), has tall narrow spikes with every heartbeat from the electrical signal going through the ventricles to make the muscle squeeze. I asked him to describe what the waveform looked like between those spikes. That's where there are small bumps in the waveform when the atria squeeze. He said the waveform looked jagged, like a "sawtooth." This is the exact description we learn in medical training for *atrial flutter* or *fibrillation* (AF or AFib). He was a smart engineer but not a physician, so it was amazing to hear him describe this over the phone. He'd just diagnosed himself—the flutter waves he described means the atria are beating faster and in a less effective way—more quivering than contracting. This means the blood doesn't flow as well through the atria, and when blood moves slowly, it can form clots.

We now knew the most likely reason he had a brief stroke, or *transient ischemic attack* (TIA), which occurs when the symptoms go away the same day. He had a heart rhythm that causes blood clots to form in the heart chamber that can go to the brain. The treatment he needed to prevent another, potentially larger, stroke was to be put on an intravenous blood thinner right away. My initial efforts to get him back to the hospital for this didn't work, likely because I was a cardiology fellow calling all the way from Boston. Thankfully, we found a physician who'd admit him and start the blood thinners. From there, they did an echocardiogram and found the underlying source of his heart disease—an abnormal heart valve that can develop years after getting rheumatic fever as a child from a strep infection. The valve was thickened and did not open fully and is a common cause of AFib. The scarred valve, together with the AFib, carries a high risk of blood clots and explains his stroke. Thankfully, with the blood thinner and careful follow-up care, he did well without any more strokes.

As you can tell from the story, his AFib was silent. While many people feel the palpitations of the heart beating quickly and irregularly with AFib, many don't. For some reason, people's sensitivity to changes in their heartbeat is different. I'm one of the sensitive types because I can feel even a single extra or skipped beat. But I've had many patients with a lot of abnormal beats during my physical examination of their heart who don't feel a thing. My wife's uncle, who had his AFib detected on a routine ECG, felt no different than before. What also makes AFib hard to detect early is that it can begin with only short episodes (what we call *paroxysmal AFib*), even when we sleep. Like heart artery plaques that can be silent until we have a heart attack, AFib can cause no symptoms until we have a stroke.

One of my patients had this exact scenario. He'd been doing well for years after a heart attack, with his plaque risk factors under control. Then, he had two mild strokes where the cause was not found. His heart rhythm was normal during the time he was monitored in the hospital. Even the usual home ECG monitor, the 24-hour Holter, hadn't picked up anything concerning.

Thankfully, a new monitor was developed by a company that came out of the Stanford Biodesign educational program mentioned earlier, codeveloped by physician-entrepreneurs Josh Makower and Paul Yock. The program has its fellows develop ideas and products for unmet medical needs. In this case, the medical need was a better way to capture intermittent heart rhythms, like AFib. One of the Biodesign teams created a small adhesive patch (*Zio patch*), like a big Band-Aid, that could be worn on the chest to record an ECG for two weeks before being simply mailed back (see FHDLC.info/Zio).[42] Instead of having only 24 hours of ECG data, there were 14 days of data to be analyzed for heart rhythm changes. This patch worked great for my patient and caught his silent AFib episodes. This let us put him on the right blood thinner to prevent future strokes.

This type of heart monitoring has now been integrated into a smartwatch, a technology I've worked on at Google and Fitbit (see FHDLC .info/WatchECG)[43,44] and that we've reviewed in the *Journal of the American College of Cardiology*.[45] This is an early highlight of the growing opportunities to use mobile and digital technologies to improve health. Chapter 13 is dedicated to digital health.

Failing Heart

I'm not a big fan of the term *heart failure*. Clearly, it developed in an era of medicine when we didn't consider how it would be understood by patients or other doctors. No one wants to think that the organ that must pump all the time to keep us alive has failed. Also, the term doesn't tell us much about *why* the heart is struggling and can distract us from discovering and treating the underlying cause.

Heart failure, admittedly, is a scary term. It means that the heart is struggling to keep up with the work it must do to pump enough blood to the body. Like a traffic jam, the blood trying to flow through the heart commonly gets "backed up." This means higher pressure in the veins bringing blood to the heart. This higher pressure forces fluid to seep out of the veins and into the surrounding tissues, most commonly the lungs and legs. This fluid accumulation is *edema* or *congestion*, so we call this *congestive heart failure* (CHF). When CHF develops, it must be taken seriously because the prognosis can be worse than many cancers.

I first met one of my now longtime clinic patients when he came into the hospital because he couldn't breathe. His echocardiogram showed that his heart wasn't squeezing well, causing fluid buildup in his lungs—a classic presentation of CHF. But what started it? Why didn't his heart squeeze normally? The most common cause of CHF is a heart attack, which kills heart muscle cells so we don't have enough muscle to squeeze well enough to meet the body's demands. This becomes another big reason to prevent plaque buildup and heart attacks, because even if you survive a heart attack, the damage may result in CHF, which can become a lifelong battle. While there are now interventions that can improve heart failure, such as drugs, artificial pumps, and heart transplant, CHF remains a top cause of having to go to the hospital. Five-year mortality approaches 50% for many groups of patients, similar or worse than many cancers. I refer you to the elegant writing of Sandeep Jauhar, a cardiologist who specializes in heart failure, and his book *Heart: A History* for a more extensive discussion of the failing heart.[46]

The good news in my patient's case was that the ECG and blood tests didn't show a heart attack. When we saw that his blood pressure was high in the hospital, we didn't think much about it given the stress of the event. In talking to him more, I learned that he'd been told a while back that he had high blood pressure but hadn't followed up with a doctor for years. We'll talk in more detail about the "silent killer" of high blood pressure as a major contributor to heart attacks, strokes, and heart failure. In his case, all that time with high blood pressure caused his heart muscle to weaken from the extra work. In the hospital, we could give him medications to remove the extra fluid in his lungs and bring his blood pressure down. This helped his heart pump more efficiently. The real questions were: What would happen when he went home? Would he get serious about his heart health or succumb to the cancer-like poor prognosis of CHF? Thankfully, as you may have guessed from his introduction as a "longtime" patient, he's been great about taking his blood pressure medications, improving his exercise and diet (see the section on "suicide foods"), and coming to see me in clinic. With all this, his heart muscle function improved back to normal, and he hasn't had heart failure since!

Bulging Vessels

While we've focused on plaque tumor buildup in our arteries as the main cause of heart attacks and strokes, I'd be remiss if I didn't highlight the opposite problem of bulging arteries, called *aneurysms*. You may have heard of the ESPN reporter, Grant Wahl, dying suddenly at the 2022 World Cup from a ruptured aortic aneurysm. Most aneurysms like his have a genetic cause and are inherited, like the well-known *Marfan syndrome*. The aorta, near where the coronary arteries emerge, becomes enlarged over time and its wall becomes thin and prone to rupture, which is often lethal. Before the advent of more rapid CT scanners, echo specialists like me would be called into the emergency room for chest pain patients to evaluate their aorta when a tear or rupture was suspected. We use a special transesophageal echo probe that can be passed into the swallowing tube (esophagus) close to the aorta, allowing us to get detailed pictures. Screening patients with a family history of aortic aneurysm or Marfan syndrome is important to detect an aneurysm before it gets too large and prone to rupture because the aneurysm can be surgically replaced to prevent rupture.

My father had the other main type of aortic aneurysm—an *abdominal aortic aneurysm* (AAA)—a bulge in the aorta as it goes behind the stomach and continues down to supply the legs. AAAs mostly occur in older people and share many risk factors with plaque buildup, including age, male sex, cigarette smoking, high blood pressure, and high cholesterol. We've mentioned that inflammation is a big contributor to plaque growth, and we and others have found that it also contributes to AAA growth.[47,48] Fortunately, studies have shown that screening for those at risk for AAA can save lives. An abdominal ultrasound can provide early detection of AAAs and then regular monitoring, like with my dad. In the United States, the Medicare health plan covers AAA screening when someone joins at 65, so check if you or a family member qualifies (see FHDLC.info/AAAscreen).[49]

CHAPTER 7

Cancer and Heart Disease Intertwined

With heart disease and cancer enveloping my family, professional and personal were now fully intertwined. Looking back at when I started telling my patients that they should think of heart disease like cancer, was I justified in scaring them that way? How similar are they really? It turns out a lot more than you'd think.

Earlier I described my introduction to cancer when I was in college, having lost my grandfather before I graduated. I honestly didn't learn much about cancer at that time other than it had taken over his body, and it was too late to do anything about it. Then my sister and I both had malignant melanomas. This sounded scary at the time, but we were lucky that, as a skin cancer, it was visible and caught early so that surgery could treat it successfully. I did learn how seriously cancer doctors approach diagnosis and care, with an attentive and careful review of the diagnosis, treatment approaches, and the likelihood of success. While cancer is almost as common as heart disease, it's still approached as a rare occurrence—which makes sense. While many people get cancer, for an individual, it's still a surprise and a life-altering event. I was beginning to see the many benefits of treating health conditions more like cancer.

My grandfather's cancer and my sister's second cancer were, in many ways, more typical—it grew inside their bodies so they couldn't easily see it forming and didn't cause symptoms until later. We described a similar issue with heart disease—plaques grow inside the heart arteries and can become life-threatening before causing symptoms. But science shows many more similarities between heart disease and cancer—not only those under the microscope, but risk factors, screening, treatment, and even prevention.[50–52]

Shared Risk Factors

At the outset of the book, one of the questions I posed was about heart disease and cancer sharing many risk factors. While I was aware of all the heart disease risk factors, I was surprised that cancer shared so many (see FHDLC.info/SharedRisk).[53] These shared risk factors are key contributors to tissue injury and inflammation, and chronic inflammation promotes growth of heart disease and cancer. Cigarette smoking is obvious because hopefully everyone is aware that it's a major contributor to heart disease and cancer, and not just lung cancer. Dietary choices are well known to contribute to heart disease and underlying problems like high blood cholesterol, blood pressure, and diabetes. But unhealthy diets also increase the risk for cancer. Promoting physical activity for heart disease prevention is near and dear to me. I've studied the benefits of physical activity using technologies from MRI to mobile devices, but the most interesting recent data show that physical activity can prevent many types of cancer. Indeed, the scientists reviewing the data for the 2018 update to the official Physical Activity Guidelines for Americans devoted an entire chapter to the types of cancer physical activity can help prevent.[54] Obesity, which emerged rapidly as the major noncommunicable pandemic of this century, is now the second leading *modifiable* risk factor for cancer![55] Don't forget alcohol. Excess consumption is associated with increased heart disease, and any consumption with breast, colon, liver, and other cancers. While these shared risk factors indicate similarities in the causes of heart disease and cancer, optimistically, they also provide the opportunity for shared prevention. We'll get to that later.

Intertwined Biology and Therapy

We've considered how Virchow, in the 1800s, found atheroma to be active growths with inflammation, a feature he also found in cancer. He was the first to find that contributors to chronic inflammation can promote both heart disease and cancer. In general, inflammation is helpful as it's a way that our immune system fights disease. But too much inflammation, or ongoing, chronic inflammation, can impact our healthy tissues. What do we know about inflammation in the malignant coronary plaques we've been discussing? The main culprit is the *macrophage* (macro=big, phage=eat), a special form of white blood cell that's normally beneficial. It not only helps fight infection, but also clears out diseased tissue. In the setting of the various risk factors we've described, macrophages enter the vessel wall, but some die and attract more, accumulating and causing plaques to grow and develop the inflamed "pus" Virchow described. The malignant aspect is that macrophages can break down the sturdy part of the plaque and cause it to crack or rupture. This triggers the clot formation that blocks blood flow and causes a heart attack.

How do macrophages relate to cancer? They typically target diseased tissue, including cancer cells. But cancer cells can mimic healthy tissue to avoid macrophages. To protect themselves, healthy cells put a protein on their surface to tell macrophages, "don't eat me." Cancer cells, to avoid attack by immune cells, often express this protective protein. Scientists have developed cancer drugs to "hide" the "don't eat me" protein from macrophages, allowing them to kill the cancer cells. Colleagues at Stanford thought that plaque tumors could have the same issue, preventing macrophages from doing their usual beneficial job of clearing diseased tissue from the artery wall. First, they found that plaques had much more of the "don't eat me" protein than usual. When they gave animals the same anticancer drug to block the protective protein, it helped macrophages reduce plaque buildup! Plaques were indeed behaving like cancer, with this novel anticancer therapy allowing macrophages to fight rather than promote heart disease.[56]

Another hallmark of cancer now found to be active in heart disease is *angiogenesis*, the term for the body growing (-genesis) new blood vessels (angio-). This sounds like a good thing for heart disease. When there are blockages in the heart arteries due to advanced plaque buildup, angiogenesis helps by forming small new arteries that improve blood supply. Good. In cancer, however, angiogenesis is a major problem because it allows tumors to increase the blood supply they need to grow. Bad. Angiogenesis can be bad in heart disease too. As plaques grow in the artery wall, they, like tumors, send out signals to grow more small blood vessels to keep feeding the plaque and help it grow. These new (neo) vessels are leaky and fragile, facilitating the entry of inflammatory and red blood cells into the plaque, making it more inflamed and likely to cause heart attacks.

It was a surgeon in Boston, Judah Folkman, who first hypothesized that angiogenesis was key to cancer tumor growth with an article in the *New England Journal of Medicine* in 1971.[57] He observed that growing tumors had more blood vessels and that certain tumors remained limited in size when blood vessel growth was limited. He then showed in the laboratory that experimental tumors in animal models could stimulate new vessels in as little as six hours! Thinking there had to be a molecule released by tumors that triggered this blood vessel growth, he coined the term *anti-angiogenesis* as a new approach to cancer treatment. While it took many years to find these pro-angiogenesis molecules and then anti-angiogenesis drugs, there are now over a dozen angiogenesis inhibitors for cancer therapy.[58]

When I first learned about angiogenesis and heart disease, it was the engineering approach—how to provide more pipes to supply blood flow to the heart. We knew from coronary angiograms that the body could form new blood vessel branches when there was a severe blockage. Dr. Folkman's work had led to the discovery of pro-angiogenesis molecules and the initial thought was to use them to increase the blood supply in patients with advanced heart disease, beyond what a stent or bypass surgery could. Unfortunately, no clear clinical benefit has emerged yet from this approach. Another cardiology fellow in Boston, Karen Moulton, introduced me to the concept of anti-angiogenesis for heart disease. While I was researching imaging of diet interventions on plaque growth, she was doing research with Dr. Folkman. As mentioned, pathological examination of plaques had shown small vessels growing in them, with more advanced, malignant plaques having more neo vessels. This similarity to Dr. Folkman's findings with cancer tumors led to the idea that inhibiting new vessel growth into plaques could prevent plaque growth. Drs. Moulton, Folkman, and colleagues tested several new anti-angiogenesis drugs in animal models and showed that they reduced plaque growth by 70%–85% without changing cholesterol levels.[59] Research on using anti-angiogenesis cancer drugs to combat plaque buildup continues, though not in time to help Dr. Folkman, who died of a heart attack. A major challenge is the two sides to angiogenesis and how to promote or inhibit it only in the location needed. Delivery of these drugs throughout the body can have unintended consequences on cancer or the heart (see later chapter on cardiooncology). This research has helped the plaque imaging field, and I integrated angiogenesis imaging into my research, as we'll discuss.

Now let's talk about one of the most recent, and closest, links between cancer and heart disease. You're likely familiar with how cancer cells are called *clones*—they grow by making copies of themselves. My younger sister and father were both diagnosed with a form of cancer (chronic lymphocytic leukemia) where there are many clones of the infection-fighting white blood cells circulating or collecting in lymph nodes. Many more people than we realized have clones of white blood cells circulating, but at a lower, pre-cancerous level. This finding, what could be considered pre-leukemia, is now recognized as a cause of heart attacks. Dr. Peter Libby, whom I cited earlier as a leader in rediscovering the role of inflammation in plaque development, has also written about this *clonal hematopoiesis*, or CHIP.[60] While he acknowledges that this "differs from cancer," it can be considered "one step down the path to leukemia." This newly discovered blood marker confers a 40%

increase in heart disease risk beyond traditional risk factors! This is a dramatic example of how heart disease and cancer are intertwined, where analyzing the blood for cancer changes may be just as important for heart disease prediction and prevention.

Imaging Plaque "Biology"

Not surprisingly, if our understanding of heart disease was evolving, imaging needed to evolve too. In earlier chapters, we talked about how we'd started using MRI to see the heart arteries and if they were narrowed. Then we realized that a plaque can grow in the wall before it narrows the artery, so we needed to image the "iceberg" under the surface. We developed MRI techniques to image the plaque directly (that is, to see the coronary wall where plaques grow, not just the lumen where the blood flows above the plaque).

Now with all the science around inflammation being critical to plaque growth and vulnerability, intertwined with cancer science and the roles of macrophages and angiogenesis, we realized that we needed to image plaque *biology*. Seeing plaque in the wall was important, but even more important was knowing whether it was biologically active (malignant) or inactive (benign). When pathologists look closely, most people develop some plaque—recall that it was common in the hearts of young US soldiers killed in Vietnam. The bigger question is whether it's prone to burst and cause a heart attack. To image this biology, my research shifted to *molecular imaging*—using techniques to image the molecules and cells within tissue.

My work in molecular imaging of plaques began with MRI and what we call *magnetic nanoparticles*. A nanometer is very small—one-billionth of a meter—much smaller than the average cell. Nanoparticles, then, are very small particles, and when they're injected into the bloodstream, they circulate throughout the body. They can be equipped with imaging capabilities so we can detect where they go and accumulate.

Not surprisingly, macrophages like to ingest nanoparticles. "Cleaning up" and removing foreign substances is part of their job. We just needed a way to image these tiny particles by MRI. Not surprisingly, iron shows up on MRI. You may have had a science class in which the teacher placed a magnet near some iron particles to show how they moved in response. Because MRI uses a powerful magnet to make images, having nanoparticles made of iron is a great way to see them. We also used MRI of iron in my clinical "day job"—imaging hearts with MRI scanners in the hospital to detect heart disease. Several diseases can result in iron buildup in our organs, including the heart. Knowing this is happening in the heart can guide treatment to remove iron from the blood and prevent or reverse heart damage. The MRI signal's sensitivity to iron allows the noninvasive detection of the iron level in the heart rather than using an invasive catheter to biopsy the heart muscle. In one form of severe anemia, where frequent blood transfusions often result in iron overload, MRI has had a profound role. When the United Kingdom made MRI evaluation of iron in the heart standard for these patients to guide therapy, their rate of dying from iron overload and heart disease fell by 70%![61]

So, we and other researchers started by showing that the two ideas worked together—macrophages did indeed ingest these iron-containing nanoparticles and could be detected by MRI.[62] The next question was: would this work for imaging the macrophages in plaques to learn if a plaque was inflamed and, thus, malignant? We also wanted a nanoparticle that could be tried in humans one day. We collaborated with a research group at Montana State University who had been studying "bio-inspired" nanoparticles that different organisms make naturally. For example, viruses make protein cages or shells on the outside with their genetic material (RNA or DNA) on the inside. While this protein cage is not infectious because it doesn't have the RNA or DNA, it still didn't seem wise to use this for humans. We've become sensitized about viruses and potential pandemics, so in retrospect, this was a good decision. It turns out that the body already makes a protein cage to carry iron! The protein is called *ferritin* and its 24 subunits are precisely organized to form a tiny protein nanocage. Thus, we could use a naturally occurring human nanoparticle already designed to hold iron as our magnetic nanoparticle. Thankfully, when we created plaques in a small-animal model, we found that MRI could detect the nanoparticles in them, corresponding to the macrophages, or inflammation, providing a biological indicator of high-risk, malignant plaques.[63]

Because there are a lot of macrophages in the body, we wanted to go a step further to image not just any macrophage, but those that were "activated" and contributing most to inflammation. Another lab at Stanford realized that fireflies have this property—they have a gene that, when activated, turns on an internal light so they can be seen.[64] This lab helped develop mice with the firefly gene so its cells would light up. We asked if we could apply this to plaque macrophages—were there specific mice engineered with the firefly gene so that only cells involved in inflammation would glow? Indeed, there were, and when we created plaques in these mice and imaged them inside a dark box to pick up the light from glowing cells, we could detect active plaque inflammation noninvasively.[65]

Another approach was to enhance the nanoparticles by attaching a molecule that targets both active inflammation and angiogenesis. We discussed that growing plaques need to form new vessels, and prior research had found that certain molecules would bind to them. So, we took the protein nanocages with the iron inside (our magnetic nanoparticles) and added this angiogenesis-targeting molecule on the outside. Now our MRI technique could also detect angiogenesis in plaques.[47]

Imaging Heart Disease like an Oncologist

Our quest to detect malignant plaques was similar, in some ways, to the challenges oncologists face when taking care of a cancer patient. How do you know if a tumor is benign or malignant without having to take a tissue sample? If you underwent chemotherapy, how can you tell if the cancer cells were killed? Cancer specialists and radiologists had already made great strides on this. The main imaging technology for this is *positron emission tomography* (PET), which uses special radioactive chemicals injected into the bloodstream that emit a radioactive signal (*positron*), which is captured by a machine to generate an image (*tomogram*). Because nothing else in the body emits a radioactive signal, this technique can pick up even the smallest areas of accumulation. It's good for seeing small tumors, so maybe it could image even smaller coronary plaques.

The most common chemical used in PET imaging for cancer is *fluorodeoxyglucose* (FDG), which is like glucose, the main sugar cells take in for energy. Cells think it's glucose and bring it in like a Trojan horse carrying radioactivity, but they can't use it like glucose, so it builds up inside them. Because malignant cancer cells are growing and dividing more than normal cells, they need a lot of glucose, so a lot of FDG builds up. FDG is made radioactive and injected so the PET scan shows where cancer is growing.

I also learned about how oncologists used PET imaging from how they were following my sister's ovarian cancer. They used it initially to locate her growing tumors to guide surgery and chemotherapy. Then they followed blood markers. As you may recall, my father-in-law had helped develop many advances in the blood tests for cancer markers, including CA-125. Whenever my sister's CA-125 level went up, even a little, they checked the PET scan to catch any recurrent tumor early. Her blood test went up slightly after a year, but the scan remained negative. A year later, her CA-125 went up further, and this time, her PET scan showed two small tumors, successfully removed with another surgery.

You can probably guess what other tumors are growing with cells hungry for glucose. Malignant plaques! Remember we said that plaques with a lot of macrophages causing inflammation are at high risk for causing heart attacks? Research studies were starting to show that PET using FDG, the glucose Trojan horse for cancer imaging, could also detect inflamed plaques, even in the larger branches of the coronary arteries.[66] With FDG and PET already in clinical use for cancer, this was a promising approach because it can take many years to get a new imaging agent (like the protein nanocages) approved. There were still some major challenges to getting good PET images of plaques in the heart arteries. Not only are coronary plaques very small, they also—unlike cancer—move with every heartbeat. The first approach we explored was combining PET with my favorite—MRI—because there were new PET/MRI scanners to provide the benefits of both. MRI was good at seeing the heart arteries and where plaque was building up in the artery walls, while PET using FDG was good at picking up the active macrophages in plaque inflammation. The combination was also important because MRI could improve the PET image, like how the motion stabilizers on your phone's camera help take sharper pictures. Having the MRI also track heart motion could adjust the PET image accordingly, making small inflamed plaques more visible. Maybe PET/MRI could do for heart disease what it does for oncology. It could show when plaques are active and need more aggressive therapy but also when they're inactive to let us know that treatment is working.

One of the smart research fellows in my lab had the idea to add this biological or molecular imaging capability to the end of a catheter. Recall that cardiologists use catheters to inject dye into the coronary arteries to see blockages and guide where to put a stent or do bypass surgery. We talked about how Paul Yock added ultrasound to the end of a catheter to see how much plaque was growing in the wall, even in arteries without significant narrowing. What was still missing was whether these plaques were biologically active. A severe blockage may warrant a stent to improve blood flow, but if we could detect malignant plaques not causing blockages, could stenting them prevent heart attacks? Dr. Raiyan Zaman figured out how to create a catheter PET scanner. She put a sensor at the end of a fiberoptic catheter so that it could convert the radioactive signal from FDG into light. Then the light could pass along the fiberoptic catheter to a camera. This allowed up-close imaging of plaque inflammation with the goal of guiding cardiologists during the procedure so they know which plaques are malignant, close to bursting, and in need of treatment.[67–69] This is another opportunity for cardiologists to learn how to image heart disease like an oncologist!

CHAPTER 8

Prevention over Imaging

Just as I was getting deeper into the application of cancer imaging to coronary plaques, my career shifted focus again because of what I was encountering with my patients. My clinical practice had moved toward a focus on prevention. I had the privilege of taking on the directorship of Stanford's Preventive Cardiology Clinic, one of the first in the country to show that improving lifestyle and controlling risk factors could reduce risk of a heart attack.[70] My goal in developing imaging technologies to detect coronary plaques before they caused heart attacks was—to prevent heart attacks! Imaging without the prevention wouldn't accomplish anything. What became clearer in talking with my patients is that they struggled to do all those healthy, preventive things, which we'll dive into further with AHA's Life's Essential 8. I realized that my research on multimillion-dollar PET/MRI scanners to see malignant coronary plaques may help someday, but the bigger challenge and opportunity in front of me was helping more people with prevention. That's what really needed to happen—at the individual level to help my patients and at population scale to address the "pandemic" of heart disease in the United States and growing around the world.

Health Happens Every Day

The other major realization to come from my clinic patients, as both a failing of our medical school teaching and a major opportunity for prevention, is that health doesn't happen in an MRI scanner. Health happens every day, outside the "four walls" of a medical building. The basic daily choices we make about being physically active and, more importantly, what we put in our mouths—from foods to drinks to cigarettes to medications—determine our health over the long term. They contribute to all the risk factors we described and the heart disease (and even cancer) that can follow. In talking with patients about improving these behaviors, I realized that I'd never learned anything about behavior in medical school. I learned everything about the myriad diseases we can succumb to and their underlying biology, appearance under the microscope, signs and symptoms, diagnostic tests, and treatments. But fundamental to preventing these diseases is behavior. There's actually a whole field of behavioral science, including behavioral medicine. Physicians have a unique opportunity to help patients improve their health, but we never learned the science behind behavior and how to help people make better, healthier choices.

One aspect of behavior I learned firsthand is people are often more motivated to change their lifestyle for their families than for themselves. I met one of my patients when he learned that he and his wife needed to take over care of their granddaughter. At that time in his life, he had high blood pressure (hypertension), diabetes, and obesity—for a cardiologist, a ticking time bomb. Worse, at his last primary care visit, his diabetes was out of control and insulin injections were recommended. The thought of his worsening condition when he needed to be there for his granddaughter helped him rethink his daily choices. He got a pedometer—this was before smartwatches—to get 10,000 steps in per day and changed his diet. Over time, his hypertension, diabetes, and weight all improved so much that he was able to maintain both his blood pressure and glucose at healthy levels without medications!

His improved daily habits and staying on his cholesterol medication for the past 20 years has kept him heart attack free. More importantly, unlike my father-in-law, he's been there for his granddaughter, who's now all grownup.

Health and Research Go Mobile

The other big change that occurred after I started directing the Stanford Preventive Cardiology Clinic was the birth of *mobile health*. Mobile phone use was growing rapidly, and companies were including miniaturized sensors in mobile devices, from phones to wearables. A large proportion of the world's population now had computers and sensors in their hands. Remember our discussion about health relating to daily behaviors and decisions? The challenge for medicine has been that these behaviors were going unmeasured. How can we help people with their daily health if we can't help them measure and improve? What better platform than devices we interact with many hours per day, mostly to connect with our friends and family? What an opportunity to use these mobile devices for health promotion!

Heart disease was especially relevant for mobile health because devices were beginning to measure everything from physical activity to heart rate, blood pressure, and even an ECG. This emerging science completed the transition of my clinical and research focus from imaging to mobile health as the best way to promote prevention. Here was an opportunity for technology to capture daily "snapshots" of health with devices that were accessible to most (not all—more on that later). I then helped the AHA bring together physicians, nurses, scientists, and companies large and small to an inaugural "Health Tech" forum in 2014 in Austin, TX, which led to our publishing the first "roadmap" for cardiovascular mobile health.[71]

Then Apple called. They wanted to enable the use of their phones for heart disease research. They were developing software that would let people participate in a research study through their phones without having to come into a hospital or clinic. What a great way to study heart health and prevention at scale! We called the study MyHeart Counts and used the phone's sensors to measure daily physical activity and do a fitness test (see FHDLC.info/MyHeartCounts).[72] The US recommendations for physical activity at the time were based on research studies using surveys, which are imprecise. In MyHeart Counts, we could measure physical activity throughout the day, including estimates of how intensely we walk or jog, because intensity has been more strongly associated with health benefit and longevity than the total amount of activity. For the fitness assessment, we replicated a standard clinical test that measures how far you can walk in six minutes. Finally, we gave people the opportunity to get their heart disease risk score through their phone, calculated per AHA guidelines, and with this estimate their "heart age."

When the MyHeart Counts study launched in 2015 with four other studies, the enrollment exceeded our most optimistic predictions. Ten thousand participants enrolled in the first 24 hours and 50,000 in the first few months.[73] This made it clear that mobile devices built for consumers rather than medical devices built for patients were the way to reach a large population. Consumer companies, who understood people's daily needs and wants much better than the medical community, were better positioned to do this. That's why I chose to take a leave from my Stanford professorship and join Google later that year.

Reengineering Health Care

These rapid-fire experiences—the importance of daily decisions in health, the idea that most health takes place outside the hospital, the birth of mobile health, and the potential for consumer devices and tech companies to advance health at scale—all called for "reengineering" our approach to health care. This has been my main career driver over the last decade. Health care naturally developed around helping people when they get sick by figuring out what the problem is and providing treatment. That's the bulk of what we're taught in medical school, and that's where most health care dollars are spent. Many people have re-named this "sick" care. We all want great care when we're sick. What's been hard for the health care system is also providing great preventive care—"health" care. As we've discussed, prevention is a daily thing and includes daily choices about activity and nutrition, blood pressure and blood sugar levels, remembering to take medications, and so on. Our health care system, which is based on you, the patient coming to us, the clinicians is not designed to help every day. I usually start con-versations around this with the mental exercise of how you'd want to reengineer health care from scratch. You'd want it to come to you, to help you with those daily behaviors and measurements, to monitor your status regularly, to catch changes early before you get sick, and to be available to all. Even if you got sick and had to go to the hospital, you'd like to get back home soon and allow careful monitoring of recovery there so you don't have to go back. This sounds like putting you—the person, not the doctor or hospital—at the center of "health" care. How could we flip the model to design *patient-centered care* (an idea the cardiologist Eric Topol captures well in the title of his book, *The Patient Will See You Now*)?[74] Later, we'll go into all the work on leveraging advances in computers, sensors, data science, artificial intelligence, and so on—what has gone from being called mobile health to *digital health*. I've dedicated an entire chapter to this. First, let me follow through on making you the center of health and care and empower you with the essential information to help yourself and your loved ones.

Turning Heart Disease Benign

I hope you've learned a lot by this point, and I'm overdue to help you turn this new knowledge into action. The key message is to take a new perspective on heart disease based on the science and the seriousness of its consequences—namely to think about and fight it as you would cancer. How can you use this new knowledge and understanding to help your health or that of family or friends? How can a modern view that heart disease is like cancer and should be treated like it help you?

I've mapped out the combination of the prevention, screening, and treatment approaches of a cardiologist *and* an oncologist. How do you avoid getting heart disease (and cancer at the same time)? How do you check if you have risk factors and which ones you can improve? How do you screen for early disease before you get symptoms (or worse)? What's the best therapy to keep or turn heart disease benign?

I'd love to say curing heart disease is simple, but it's not. As you can tell from my family stories, even having a preventive cardiologist in the family can only help so much. So, while I want to empower you with the knowledge to help, don't take on all of the burden yourself. As with cancer, involvement of family and friends can be a tremendous support. And you should expect your health care provider to step up to assist you and take your heart health as seriously as cancer. So, let's learn the key ways to prevent you from getting tumors in your heart arteries, screen to find them early when you're at risk, and treat them so they don't turn malignant. *Let's prevent, screen, and treat heart disease like cancer.*

CHAPTER 9

Prevent Like It's Cancer

Prevention is obviously a great place to start. The core elements for preventing heart disease are helpful at every stage of life and every stage of disease. That's why, as a preventive cardiologist, I think of everyone as my patient! These tools help young and old avoid risk factors, prevent risk factors from turning into heart disease, prevent heart disease from causing heart attacks, and if you've had a heart attack, prevent another.

We discussed how heart disease and cancer share many risk factors, so you likely aren't surprised that many of the top prevention actions work for both. I must admit that before I wrote this book, I hadn't realized that the prevention websites for the AHA and the American Cancer Society (ACS) had so much in common. The four preventable risk factors these websites share are to move more, eat healthy, manage weight, and avoid tobacco—all in the AHA's Life's Essential 8 and the ACS's prevention guidelines (see FHDLC.info/AHAessential8 and FHDLC.info/ACSprevention).[75,76]

Because I'm a longtime supporter and volunteer for the AHA, it will also not surprise you that the prevention advice here is based on AHA's Life's Essential 8 but with a twist. In thinking more like an oncologist, I've carved three out from the eight and moved them into the next chapter ("Screen Like It's Cancer"). These other three essential steps involve controlling blood cholesterol, blood pressure, and blood glucose, but they require screening first because many people don't know when they have abnormal levels putting them at risk. These conditions also often need treatment beyond diet and exercise to get and keep these growth factors under control. More to come.

When I started this book, the AHA's program was called Life's Simple 7. It was developed as part of the AHA's 2010 publication setting out the AHA Impact Goal for 2020.[77] This was a milestone because the prior AHA goals focused on reducing the bad outcomes of heart disease and not on increasing heart health. The AHA developed this measure of heart health to track "cardiovascular health promotion *and* disease reduction." These seven were the four prevention steps shared with the ACS and the three just mentioned (blood cholesterol, blood pressure, and blood glucose). I'll go into the first four in more depth in this chapter plus the newest addition (number 8) to the AHA program—sleep. I've also added two more: alcohol and stress. We've continued to learn how they contribute to heart disease (and cancer), and they were both exacerbated by COVID-19, so they're important to include.

One last editorial comment before we dive in is that I like the change in the AHA program's name away from "simple." It's important to acknowledge that changing behaviors is more often hard than simple, and when there's a long list of things to incorporate into our daily lives, it's even less simple. Progress on any of the following items can help, so start where you can, and don't try to do it all on your own.

Move More

The "miracle drug" to prevent heart disease and many other diseases is getting and staying physically active. Studies have shown that, for every extra minute you're active, you add at least five to your life![78] That's an incredible return on investment. Also, every time there's a big review of outcomes data, we find more cancers that are prevented by physical activity. It helps our mental health, too. Heart, cancer, brain—win-win-win.[79]

We'd all like to move more, but life's busy, and it can be hard to make time. The main question is: how much physical activity do we really need for heart health and cancer prevention? The short answer is that any activity helps. The better answer is to find activities you like *and* that get your heart beating faster. The first part makes sense—if we want to integrate regular physical activity into our lives, we want to do activities we—and our bodies—like. I used to do running as 90% of my exercise. Running with my dog, Arlie, was great fun for both of us— it doesn't take much planning or equipment and gets you outdoors when the weather cooperates. Now that my knees and back have aged and Arlie turned 14, we don't run as much. Now I mix in biking and swimming—great for my joints, but not Arlie's favorites!

So, what do we mean about wanting to get our heart beating faster? That's another way of saying that we can get more "bang for the buck" if we do more moderate or vigorous activities. We now have tons of long-term data showing that "moderate-to-vigorous" activity is most helpful for living longer and disease free. While that may sound hard, it's not. The simplest moderate activity is brisk walking. This can be wherever it's easiest for you to walk on your own, with friends, or with your dog.

The other good news is that all your activities add up. The world-wide guidelines for physical activity have us add up all the minutes we do in a week, so you can do more some days and less others. The main goal is 150 minutes per week, or about 30 minutes a day, 5 days per week, and that's if you do mostly moderate activities. If you can do some vigorous activities, like jogging, lap swimming, or singles tennis, those minutes count double! The 2018 update to the US physical activity guidelines reaffirmed this. They recommend 150 or more of moderate minutes per week, or half of that (75 minutes or more per week, or 15 minutes per day) if those minutes are vigorous.[80] What can be confusing is how to keep track of these minutes. What if some are moderate and some are vigorous? Well, the guidelines give us the math—to get to the 150 minute per week target, combine your moderate minutes with double your vigorous minutes. Few people want to do math every day, so one of our projects at Google was to work with the AHA and the World Health Organization (WHO) to do the math for people. We called them Heart Points—one point for every minute of moderate activity and two for vigorous minutes, with the goal of 30 per day to get you to your weekly goal of 150 Heart Points. It used your phone or wearable device to determine your walking/jogging speed or how much your heart rate goes up to estimate your moderate and vigorous activity minutes. We did a blog post on making your Heart Points count (see FHDLC.info/HeartPoints)![81]

But what about the 10,000 steps per day goal? That sounds simpler, right? Yes and no. If you've done 10,000 steps in a day, you know that can take a while, particularly the slower you go. That number didn't come from any science. It was marketing in the 1960s to promote a Japanese pedometer. The committee that reviewed the physical activity data for updating the guidelines in 2018 didn't find enough long-term data to recommend a specific step number, but here's where the math can help again. Recall that I said a brisk walk is moderate activity, which is walking at a cadence of at least 100 steps per minute. The guidelines recommend 30 minutes per day. So, 30 minutes at 100 steps per minute multiplies to 3,000 steps per day. So, 10,000 is a great goal, but if you can get in 3,000 brisk steps (should we call these Heart Steps?), you'll get to your daily goal. Because we all have busy schedules, that's the most efficient way to go. The good news is that the more steps, minutes, or Heart Points you can do the better, but even getting halfway has proven health benefits.

What about the recent statement about sitting being the new smoking? In many ways, that's saying the same thing—lack of physical activity will increase your risk of heart disease and cancer, just like smoking cigarettes. Breaking up the amount of time you spend sitting appears to be helpful. That was one of the findings in our MyHeart Counts mobile phone study—participants who more often changed activity level throughout the day reported better health status.[73] Standing instead of sitting, or standing periodically throughout the day, however, doesn't substitute for those brisk steps or minutes of getting your heartbeat going.

Forming and keeping healthy habits can be hard, especially as we go through different life stages and unexpected disruptions like COVID-19. My daughter, Kelly, has a valuable perspective, especially given the unfavorable genes we've passed along (spoiler alert—more on our genetic risk factor to come).

> *Maintaining a healthy lifestyle has become important to me, as I have the family history of heart disease on my mom's side and a genetic risk factor inherited from my dad. My first goal towards healthy habits has been to exercise 4–5 times per week. This was easy until graduating college, as I played on organized sports teams since I was 7. I now needed to find ways to provide the structure and motivation that team sports had provided for so long. I found my solution in group workout classes that I enjoyed, helping me meet my weekly goal. The covid pandemic then forced me to reassess and adapt my routine, and find an alternative workout approach. With all that has been going on, I had to make it easy for myself mentally. This meant reducing the energy put into decision making and tying new habits to ones I've already established, favoring long-term consistency over daily perfection.*

Eat Healthy

The saying should be that unhealthy eating is the new smoking! What we eat and drink has such a huge influence on our health, yet for most people, those choices default to what is "normal" in their worlds. You may have heard the research that obesity is "contagious." Humans are social animals and want to be part of the group around them.[82] It's hard to make changes, even healthy ones, if no one else is. If everyone viewed eating a hamburger and fries as we now view smoking a cigarette, it would be a lot easier to get people to shift to healthier eating.

This is one way to reframe our choices—the idea of a "cigarette diet." If we think about eating unhealthy foods the same way we think about cigarette smoking, could that mindfulness, and caring about ourselves and others, shift our mindset?

There was a simple but seminal moment in a mobile health course we did as part of Stanford Biodesign. An executive from a large computer chip company described how the company had shifted to providing their own health insurance, so everyone's monthly premium would depend on how healthy everyone was at the company. He was getting on the elevator and someone else got on with a hamburger and fries from the cafeteria. While that was not a new occurrence, he now had a new perspective. His thought was no longer "that looks good" but "what are you doing to my health insurance premium?!"

Christopher Gardner, a colleague at Stanford who teaches nutrition, has learned that, for many people, it's better to approach nutrition health by "stealth."[83] We talked about how behavior can be hard to change, yet it's fundamental to prevention. We gravitate toward behaviors that are easy and reward us now but struggle with behaviors that are hard and reward us later. That's why "delayed gratification" is rarely our first choice, but there's a lot of evidence that it's an important skill. Some of that data comes from a study in a preschool at Stanford in the 1970s, where the children who could wait a little while to get two marshmallows did better in life than the children who opted for the one marshmallow right away.[84] Making healthy diet choices every day is not as easy as waiting a bit and getting two marshmallows. A marshmallow diet is not the solution. Framing healthy diet choices to live longer is the ultimate in delayed gratification and is not motivating for most people, especially if it's eating differently than your peers.

What did Dr. Gardner find in his nutrition class with Stanford students? They were motivated to eat a healthier, more plant-based diet (more on that later) by the most important issues to them in their present world. The "stealth" was that their own long-term health was not top of mind, but connecting a meat-based diet to climate change, drought, or animal cruelty was strong motivation to change.

Another important part of changing behaviors is that it can be hard to change everything at once. I encourage patients to start with changing one aspect of their diet and go from there. One of the first changes in our family's diet started for one of these "stealth" reasons. Mad Cow disease hit the United States in 2003. While rare, no one wanted to get a neurodegenerative disease without a cure. The United States blocked testing every cow to keep it out of the food supply, unlike Japan, so our family stopped eating beef. Once accustomed to that change, it became our new normal. We now have beef once per year—grass-fed corned beef for St Patrick's day, of course.

I've started talking about a healthy plant-based diet and the harms of meat. What is a healthy diet, anyway? As most readers will know, the science around nutrition isn't perfect. For most treatments we recommend in medicine, we have answers from double-blinded, placebo-controlled, randomized trials. That means we randomly select who gets the active treatment and who gets an inactive treatment (*placebo*) so they and their doctor can't tell which they got. That's hard to do for the foods we eat, but there have been many studies, including randomized trials, of nutrition. The author Michael Pollan has distilled the science well. What he found was that people who live long and healthy lives "eat food. Not too much. Mostly plants."[85] When you think about the risk factors for heart disease—high blood cholesterol, blood sugar, blood pressure, and weight—there is a strong match. Real food, unlike processed, is much less likely to be loaded with sugar, salt, and calories. Meat, unlike plants, drives up the bad cholesterol in our bloodstream. Large portion sizes get us on a path where physical activity can't balance enough to keep our weight in check.

Another description for a healthy plant-based diet is *Mediterranean diet*. I like this one because it goes with the image of being on an island in the Mediterranean. Actually, the famous island in that regard is Crete. Early studies of fat intake and heart disease in different countries had shown a strong positive relationship—countries with higher fat intake had higher heart disease. That was part of the data that led to the recommendation for a low-fat diet. Like many well-intentioned ideas, it had unintended consequences. Namely, more *carbohydrates* (sugars) were added to replace the fat in foods. This likely contributed to the worsening of *metabolic health* with the recent increases in obesity, diabetes, and high blood pressure. Crete was a big outlier in the data. Not only did it not fit the curve correlating high fat diets with early death, Cretans had the highest fat intake but the lowest heart disease. When their diet was investigated further, their fat came from a plant in the form of olive oil, not meat. Cretans eat a ton of olive oil—more than Italians! This is one of many examples of how we learned that plant-based fats are healthy fats.

The AHA issued a presidential advisory detailing this, based on the latest science and clinical studies on dietary fat and heart disease.[86] The consistent finding is that replacing saturated with unsaturated fat in the diet lowered bad cholesterol and heart disease. Clinical trials that replaced saturated fat with carbohydrates did not show this benefit. So, what are sources of healthy fats? There are many, including canola oil, olive oil, peanuts, almonds, avocados, and fish. *Saturated fats* are primarily from animal sources—butter, lard, pork, beef, and so on. Beware of tropical oils, such as palm and coconut oils, which are high in saturated fat. I'm aware of this because, in our plaque imaging research, we used coconut oil to simulate a "Western" diet. In animal models, this causes high cholesterol and rapid plaque buildup. This also highlights that, counterintuitively, our blood cholesterol level is more related to the types of fat than the amount of cholesterol in our food.

Replacing saturated fats with simple carbohydrates is not helpful because it can negatively impact our metabolic health, but replacing saturated fat with whole grains is beneficial. As there are "healthy fats," there are "healthy carbs" in the form of whole grains. Going to a strict low-carb diet can have adverse health consequences, depending on the foods you eat to replace the carbs. I've had several patients try "paleo" diets—meant to replicate what humans ate in the Stone Age—or a similar low-carb "keto" diet. On the positive side, it encourages unprocessed "real food" (per Michael Pollan's book), but on the flip side, it encourages high meat consumption (even though access to meat was limited in the Stone Age). I've seen some patients double their bad cholesterol (!) on a paleo diet, which thankfully returned to normal when they went back to a plant-based diet.

There are, of course, many promising areas of research on diet and heart disease. One is modifying the timing of eating through *intermittent fasting*. There's strong evidence in animal studies, plus shorter-term data in humans, that time-restricting eating or fasting several days per week has beneficial effects on markers of metabolic health and inflammation, contributors to heart disease and cancer.[87] However, a year-long study of obese patients showed no benefit on weight loss or heart disease risk factors.[88] Clinical trials continue on ways to apply this promising science to improve human health. The other promising area of research relates to the *microbiome*, namely the diverse microbes that live within our gut and interact with us and the food we eat. While this is a broad field of health research, there's growing scientific evidence linking red meat consumption with a change in the microbiome that promotes heart disease. In studies led by a preventive cardiologist at Cleveland Clinic, the L-carnitine in red meat causes our microbiome to produce a chemical, *trimethylamine* (TMAO), which we absorb from our gut. TMAO promotes the malignant plaque biology we discussed— causing plaque inflammation and blood clot formation and increasing the risk for heart attacks and strokes.[89,90] Blood levels of TMAO may become a new biomarker for heart disease risk, and therapies to reduce the microbiome's production of TMAO are being tested.

The most practical, evidence-based advice I give my patients is to follow a Mediterranean diet because several randomized trials have shown a 30% or greater reduction in heart attacks, strokes, or death.[86] This diet entails replacing animal fat with healthy oils, nuts, fish, fruits, and vegetables—and tastes great! Dr. Gardner's research also shows that people are better at maintaining a Mediterranean diet than a keto diet.[91] The AHA has created a "one-pager" with guidance on creating a healthy eating pattern. Look for the AHA "heart-check" label on healthy foods and access hundreds of heart-healthy recipes (see FHDLC.info/EatHealthy).[92]

Flatten the Weight Curve

It would be overly simplistic for me to say everyone overweight should just lose weight. If weight loss were easy, we wouldn't have the obesity and metabolic health challenges facing our population. I could devote the entire book to this topic, but many others have already, so I'll keep my guidance here short. Another cardiologist who specializes in heart imaging and has the Agatston score named after him wrote *The South Beach Diet*, which encourages the healthy fats and healthy carbs approach discussed above.[93] Weight is clearly something most of my patients (and society) struggle with. Our species has been on this planet for millions of years, yet we've had the most dramatic form of human "evolution" or, you could say, "devolution" in the last few decades. Humans have become overweight or obese to a striking degree. Honestly, we don't fully understand why. There are many potential contributors—we eat more processed and less healthy food in much larger portions and spend more time driving or looking at screens than being physically active. How these trends turned into an obesity pandemic is still controversial. One thing science does tell us is that once you gain a lot of weight over time, your body fights hard to keep it. While going on a diet can help lose weight over a month or two, it's rare that substantial weight loss is maintained after a year. The yo-yo effect of repeat dieting can make things worse in the long run. In severe obesity, bariatric surgery has been the most effective therapy for sustained weight reduction with heart benefits. Now there's growing optimism for safe and effective weight-loss medications. Several emerging drugs initially developed to treat diabetes are showing promise for significant and longer-term weight loss.[94]

I ask my patients to focus more on the inputs—making the healthy changes to their eating and physical activity patterns—and less on the specific weight number as the measure of success. We know improving what we eat and how active we are will lead to improvements in blood cholesterol, blood pressure, blood sugar, and longevity, even without weight loss. These healthy changes also make us less likely to gain weight over time, so even flattening the usual upward curve of weight gain is an important benefit. As Kelly noted, the goal with forming healthy habits is long-term consistency over daily perfection.

Quit the Cigs and Vaping

This is another section I'll keep short because the guidance is clear. In many countries, public health efforts have made great progress in reducing cigarette smoking, given its strong risk for heart disease and cancer. But many people have still gotten addicted, often early in life, and it's a hard habit to break. I've had quite a few patients struggle to quit. The good news is that there are effective smoking cessation programs and medications to help. Plus, each attempt at quitting increases the chance of stopping for life.

Vaping electronic or e-cigarettes has emerged as a popular way to continue inhaling nicotine without some of the other harmful chemicals in cigarette smoke. While initially viewed as helpful to get people off cigarettes, nicotine is still a contributor to heart disease. Vaping has become an easy way for kids to get started on the habit, and it hasn't been shown to help people quit smoking in the end.[95]

The good news, as we'll discuss, is that the FDA is working to lower the addictiveness of cigarettes and vaping to get fewer hooked and help more quit. Avoiding smoking in the first place is the best way to go. Otherwise, work with your health care provider on a cessation program.

Sleep and the 24-Hour Cycle

As mentioned, the AHA has updated its prevention program to add an eighth item—healthy sleep. You already know that we (ideally) spend close to one-third of our lives asleep. It's only recently that we've started to pay more attention to its importance for health, including heart health. Getting a good night's rest helps us do many of the healthy things we discussed. It's associated with more physical activity during the day, better eating habits, and better weight control. On physical activity, the *New York Times* had an interesting discussion on which is more important: enough exercise or enough sleep (see FHDLC.info /SleepExercise).[96] The best answer I can give is that both are helpful and, as we'll discuss, each helps the other. At the end of the day (pun intended), I recommend squeezing in the 30 minutes of physical activity somewhere in your day because you have more flexibility on sleep time. Why do I say there's more flexibility for sleep? The recommended amount of sleep for adults is 7–9 hours, per the CDC, so aiming for 8 hours of sleep and fitting in 30 minutes of activity is a win-win. Plus, we have all that data on how every minute of exercise adds 5 minutes or more to our lives. Every minute of physical activity counts more than sleep, which means losing a little sleep for some exercise is the best tradeoff.

Moving during the day and sleeping at night are part of our 24-hour cycle. This means our day is a balance of active time, sedentary time, and sleep time. In the early days of wearable devices, we found that measuring active and sleep times accurately from the same device was challenging.[97] Thankfully, many wearables now help us capture how we're doing over the full 24 hours and can nudge us to get a full night's rest. It's a virtuous cycle, with more sleep helping us do more exercise and more exercise helping us sleep. Sleep also helps with multiple risk factors we'll discuss below. Not getting enough sleep can contribute to high blood pressure, diabetes, and ultimately plaque buildup.

There's another aspect of sleep and heart health to be aware of that is often unrecognized. When I was growing up, my family thought my dad was a great sleeper. He could fall asleep quickly almost anywhere, even standing up in church! But then he had a few car accidents from falling asleep on long drives to military bases for his work as a judge advocate general (JAG) in the Air Force Reserve. Sometimes I'd go with him, which I thought was a great adventure because he'd let me move the stick shift while he pushed in the clutch in our VW Squareback. But later, I learned that my mom wanted me there to keep him awake. Eventually, he was diagnosed with *sleep apnea*, which is when the throat muscles relax during sleep, narrow the airway, and obstruct breathing. Apnea means "not breathing." This can mean someone, like my dad, can be in bed for eight hours but not really get restful sleep. Even worse, when oxygen can't get into the lungs, the body reacts with a surge of *adrenaline*—our fight or flight hormone. Adrenaline increases our heart rate and blood pressure. Sleep apnea can contribute to chronic hypertension and AFib. If you have bad snoring, episodes of not breathing at night, or fall asleep too easily during the day, tell your doctor and get it checked. Sleep apnea can be treated, which helped my dad actually sleep for those recommended eight hours.

Drink Less

Humans have been consuming alcohol for 10,000 years or more. While its many harms are known, its only health benefit was thought to be for heart disease—until recently. Like many families, I grew up with the harms of alcohol. My father was an alcoholic and thankfully survived several mishaps before joining Alcoholics Anonymous and staying sober for the rest of his life. My sisters and I attended Alateen meetings and learned even more about the family harms of alcoholism. At the time, I concluded that the only way to avoid the same for my future was to avoid all alcohol, which I did all the way through college.

During medical school and cardiology training, the prevailing science was that drinking no alcohol was worse for your health than having one drink per day. The idea was that low doses of alcohol helped reduce heart disease by increasing good cholesterol (*HDL*) and reducing blood clotting. But higher doses of alcohol overwhelmed those benefits by contributing to liver disease, cancer, and other forms of heart disease. All cardiologists have seen cases of heavy drinkers where their high alcohol consumption is toxic to their heart muscle cells and causes heart failure. They've also seen patients coming to the emergency room with AFib after heavy drinking at a party (so-called "holiday heart").

During my cardiology fellowship, we did a small research study to measure those potential benefits of alcohol. We had healthy subjects drink one beer per day for a month (Sam Adams, of course, because we were in Boston). We measured changes in blood cholesterol and clotting factors. I even collaborated with my mother-in-law, Lily, on the study. She was an expert in cholesterol testing. She told us that she could run several advanced cholesterol tests on a tiny amount of blood. This was almost a decade before Theranos was founded! Of course, Lily had access to large blood-testing machines and was only testing cholesterol values, while Theranos claimed it could do many more tests on a small machine from just a drop of blood. Interestingly, we did find that this low dose of alcohol caused a significant increase in the good HDL cholesterol in both men and women, but we didn't detect a change in the blood clotting markers.[98]

How did the science change? Well, we always knew there was a big limitation to the prior data. It was epidemiology data—following people over time and cataloging their habits and how they related to future health and disease. The Framingham Study is the most powerful example of how much we can learn from epidemiologic studies, but it's always recognized that many habits go together, so an association doesn't prove causation. We'd already started to learn that clinical trials with drugs that raised HDL weren't reducing heart disease, and raising HDL was thought to be one of the main benefits of alcohol. Additional studies followed more people for longer and gathered more detailed information, which started to show no benefit to alcohol consumption. They found there were often other health issues among those who didn't drink at all that may have explained why abstinence appeared worse. Finally, genetic studies compared those with and without genes related to alcohol metabolism and consumption. This is one way to "randomize" subjects to higher and lower alcohol consumption—based on the genes they're born with. Giving them low versus high amounts of alcohol for years would be unethical. In the large UK Biobank study, an analysis led by a Stanford colleague showed that alcohol increased blood pressure and risk for stroke and AFib, plus mortality. Alcohol did not appear protective for any health condition.[99] What about the touted benefits of red wine? This is a frequent question from patients. Researchers have shown that resveratrol in red wine can help blood vessels dilate, but that's from the grape skin, not the alcohol, so simple red grape juice does the same thing.

There are no long-term randomized trials, which would be the best way to see if there's real benefit to alcohol. We don't want to promote starting alcohol consumption, because it's addictive and can have additional life and health consequences, as with my father. To top it off, studies show that alcohol increases the risk for various cancers. That's why the ACS says "it's best not to drink alcohol."[100] To prevent heart disease like cancer, the best approach to drinking is: don't start. If you already drink, try to keep it to one drink and not every day. The latest data says that limit is best for both men and women. Less is best.

Be Well

When we published the AHA's 2030 Impact Goal in 2020, a key addition was well-being as an important contributor to heart health. Well-being goes beyond physical and mental health. There are many aspects of our lives that can make us feel like we're thriving rather than struggling or suffering. You may have heard of the Gallup Poll, mostly involving political surveys. But they also have a global well-being survey, and it's been shown that lower well-being is associated with more heart disease. It's a two-way street—well-being helps heart health and a healthy heart helps well-being. We highlighted that our health care system must go beyond the traditional focus on physical health and disease and address the whole person. There's also science behind interventions to improve well-being and subsequent heart disease.[8]

How can you help yourself and those around you be well? This is an area the cancer community has understood well, with recommendations to leverage your support system of family and friends; keep a positive outlook; take care of yourself with regular physical activity and sleep; and engage in mindfulness, gratitude, and meditation. Yoga, for example, helps reduce stress through physical activity, mindfulness, and meditation, with benefits to heart disease risk factors.[101]

Like most young people these days, my daughter Kelly has had to deal with many life stressors. As a proctor in her college dormitory, she had to handle many late-night emergencies of student drug overdoses and mental health crises. She later experienced the stress and fear that developed while volunteering in a local emergency room in the early days of the COVID-19 outbreak. Her own proactive approach is one we can all learn from.

Facing a number of stressful situations in college and during the pandemic has helped me learn how to manage personal stress and it's something that I continue to consciously practice. First, I identify the stressor and try to deal with it. Is it something that is really a problem, or am I worrying unnecessarily? If the former, I try to focus on what I can control, break it down into manageable pieces, and seek help when needed. If the latter, I try to remind myself to move on. Next, I rely on my support system of friends and family. Sharing my issue helps relieve my worries and develop a plan to address it. Finally, I remind myself that taking care of myself and my immediate environment is important in minimizing additional stress. Relying on a routine that includes exercise, regular sleep, eating healthy, and organizing my surroundings helps my physical and mental health. This proactive stress management strategy, rather than trying to ignore problems, has helped me deal with many situations in a healthy manner.

One additional form of personal support that the AHA has advocated, based on science, is having a pet.[102] I mentioned Arlie as my running companion for years. He was the star of a prevention video I made when we were both able to run more (see FHDLC.info/Arlie).[103] Dogs are especially helpful for increasing physical activity, with dog owners over 50% more likely to meet the weekly physical activity recommendation. Pets also help with stress. Studies show that pet owners have lower heart rate and blood pressure responses to stressful situations, particularly when their pet is with them during the stressor. When I worked at Google before the pandemic work-from-home, taking Arlie into work once a week was a favorite activity for us. I'd make "well-being" rounds with Arlie, walking among the cubicles until, invariably, a coworker would want Arlie to hang out for a few minutes, exchanging human petting for dog licking—everyone feeling better after. You may want to try it and encourage your workplace to participate in the AHA's #BestFriendFridays for "Lots of Love. Less Stress" (see FHDLC.info/FurryFriends).[104]

Why Bother? Isn't It All in Our Genes?

Before we go to the next chapter on screening, let's talk about a common question I hear—how helpful is all this prevention given the talk about genes determining health? The short answer, and what I'm counting on for myself, is: no, it's not all in our genes. Prevention can overcome your genetic risk in most cases. I'm counting on it because I inherited a gene that increases my heart disease risk. It's *Lipoprotein(a)*, which I'll discuss later. I'm also counting on it because I've passed this gene down to Kelly and Mia.

Genetic studies do show that our genes contribute about 50% to our heart disease risk. How does that match up with what I said earlier—that heart disease is 80% preventable? Well, the good news is that there are many modifiable risk factors. While we can't (yet) change the genes we're born with, we can—through prevention, screening, and treatment—modify these risk factors to keep heart disease at bay.

Most genes found to contribute to heart disease risk each have only a small effect. Unlike with diseases such as sickle cell anemia, where a single gene causes it, most heart disease genetic risk is a combination of many risk genes. This has led to the development of "polygenic" risk scores, which we've studied in the Stanford Preventive Cardiology Clinic.[105] The hope is to ultimately combine our underlying genetic risk with the known risk factors we can measure—blood pressure, cholesterol, and glucose—to refine who needs more aggressive preventive treatment earlier in life.

While I said most heart disease genetic risk is from a combination of genes, there is one form of genetic heart disease where a single gene change can be a death sentence if not recognized and treated. At the beginning of the book, I mentioned that there are genetic mutations for heart disease just as lethal as the *BRCA* gene mutations for breast cancer, but most people affected don't know. These are mutations in genes that result in very high levels of *LDL* or bad cholesterol in our blood. This is called *familial hypercholesterolemia* (FH) and causes heart attacks. Unfortunately, it's unrecognized 80% of the time.[106] Angelina Jolie famously had a double mastectomy for her *BRCA* mutation to prevent breast cancer. For FH patients, effective prevention can be done more easily through medications to lower cholesterol to normal, which, if started early, can give them a normal lifespan. We'll talk more about screening and treating FH and Lipoprotein(a) in later chapters, but this is all the more reason to know your numbers, as we'll discuss next.

Key Takeaways: Prevention

- All physical activity helps. The more you get your heart rate going, the better. The main goal is 150 minutes per week of moderate activity (for instance, brisk walking).

- A mostly plant-based, Mediterranean diet is best to improve heart health.
- Regular physical activity and healthy eating are the best combination for weight control.
- If you smoke, get help to quit. Avoid vaping and nicotine.
- Healthy sleep promotes healthy eating and physical activity, so aim for eight hours per night.
- The latest research shows that moderate drinking does not help heart health, so less is best.
- Well-being is important for heart health, so take care of yourself and leverage your support system.
- Even if you've inherited heart disease risk, early prevention (with screening and treatment) can give you a normal lifespan.

CHAPTER 10

Screen Like It's Cancer

Does everyone need to see a preventive cardiologist? The short answer is no. Plus, there aren't enough of them to go around. But given that, currently, one of every two men and every three women get heart disease, everyone should have a preventive cardiology evaluation. Ideally, you can have your primary care provider focus on this on your next visit. Importantly, there's a lot you can do on your own or with the help of a family member to examine your heart disease risk. All the talk so far about how heart disease is like cancer won't accomplish anything unless you take this information "to heart," apply it to understanding your risk, and get help on the next steps.

How to Do a Heart "Self-Exam"

The first "screening" step is what I call a heart "self-exam." No, this doesn't require a physical exam or stethoscope to listen to your heart. As Mia described, she was taught early on the importance of self-examination and screening for breast cancer. She, like most people, didn't realize that there are self-exam tools available for heart disease for everyone to learn their risk and guide additional screening tests. There's even the equivalent of a mammogram for heart disease, which we'll get into below.

While you can use your hands to feel the heartbeat in your chest or check the pulse in your wrist or neck, that won't tell you about plaque that may be developing silently in your arteries. What can tell you a lot more is knowing your heart disease *risk score*. You actually have access to the same tool your provider is supposed to use, namely the Athero-sclerotic Cardiovascular Disease (ASCVD) risk score calculator. This score can be your self-exam, and it was developed by the AHA and the American College of Cardiology (ACC). There's also an app to make it easy to calculate your score. Now would be a great time to find it. Search on your smartphone for the "ASCVD Plus" app from the ACC, or search on the internet for the ASCVD risk calculator website (go to FHDLC.info/ASCVDrisk).[107]

What is ASCVD risk and what does it tell you and your provider? Yes, the name is a mouthful and not user-friendly. It's an example of how the health care system uses a lot of abbreviations, which makes it hard for patients to understand what's going on. ASCVD is the main theme of this book, so let me provide the translation. The CVD part is a common abbreviation for cardiovascular disease and it's what we've simply been calling heart disease. The AS part indicates *atherosclerosis*—the medical term for the plaque buildup we've been talking so much about. It comes from combining atheroma (plaque tumor) and sclerosis (hardening) to describe the changes to our arteries. Overall, our ASCVD score tells us how likely we are to have plaque buildup that will cause a heart attack, stroke, or death from heart disease.

What goes into calculating our ASCVD score and how was it developed? It started with the Framingham Heart Study. In following Framingham residents and their offspring over many years, we learned which factors were most predictive of developing heart disease. When I started in cardiology, that was the only large source of predictive data in the United States, so we were taught to use the Framingham risk score. But as we've discussed earlier, the Framingham population wasn't very diverse. Thankfully, there have been several other large studies since then following people over time, so these newer, more diverse data sets have been combined with the Framingham data to create the updated ASCVD risk score.

What information do I need to put into the ASCVD app (or website) to get my score? Yes, you need to know your numbers, as we'll go into. We mentioned that there are three other components of Life's Essential 8 for prevention—blood cholesterol, blood pressure, and blood glucose. So, beyond your age, sex, race, and smoking status, you'll need to know about those. Specifically, you need to know your cholesterol and blood pressure numbers, your diabetes status, and whether you're on medication to lower blood pressure or cholesterol. While it may take some work to track down these data, they're so important for your future health that there's a big benefit to knowing them—and getting them checked if they're not recent!

If you've run the app yourself or had it done by your provider, what do your ASCVD risk score numbers mean? The main number the app (or website) generates, if your age is between 40 and 79, is your risk for having a heart attack or stroke or dying from heart disease in the next 10 years. For example, a high ASCVD risk score is 20% or above, meaning you have more than a 1 in 5 chance of one of these events in the next 10 years. A low score is under 5%, or less than 1 in 20 chance. If your age is between 20 and 59, it will also calculate a lifetime risk for heart disease, which is going to be higher than the 10-year risk. It can be scary to look at, but it's an important indicator that none of us should ignore.

Finally, what do you do about your ASCVD risk score? This self-exam is the first step in screening for heart disease and guiding next steps. We'll go into more detail, but the high-level answer is that it lets you know if you're starting at low, moderate, or high risk. In general, a low score means the focus should be on being heart-healthy and avoiding risk factors, as we discussed in the prior chapter on prevention. A high score means you're at high risk of a malignant plaque causing a heart attack or stroke and need more aggressive therapy to stop that from happening. That's the focus of the next chapter on treatment. Note that the ASCVD risk score is for those who haven't yet had heart disease or a stroke, which would already indicate malignant plaque and mean extra focus on prevention *and* treatment to reverse the situation and avoid another event.

What about a moderate risk score between 5% and 20%? This is where it's important to take our exam to the next level. To be honest, moderate (also called intermediate) ASCVD risk tells me we don't really know whether your individual risk is low or high. It means there are some risk factors, but as I tell my patients, I can't tell from the score alone if their risk factors have added up to cause plaque buildup. I need more information to personalize your risk and care. This is also where engaging with your health care provider and shared decision making are essential because it admittedly gets complicated. The many next steps are diagrammed in Figure 3 of the heart disease prevention guidelines. [108] Importantly, there are 12 risk-enhancing factors that should be assessed, from whether you have a strong family history or high lipoprotein(a) (like me), or inflammatory conditions (such as psoriasis or HIV), or South Asian ethnicity. For many of my moderate-risk patients, I recommend an imaging test to screen for early plaque in the heart arteries as the best way to personalize care. Before we get to this mammogram for the heart, let's return to the Big Three risk factors that help us know our ASCVD risk score and are part of the AHA Life's Essential 8. We should be screening for these first.

Know Your Numbers: The Big Three

We've discussed how healthier eating and physical activity can help and are part of what I call *proactive prevention*—preventing the development of risk factors in the first place. What's the deal with those other three parts of Life's Essential 8—blood cholesterol, blood pressure, and blood sugar? Part of screening like cancer is recognizing that these are effectively growth factors for plaque—they promote the development and growth of those atheroma tumors in our coronary arteries and other vessels. They also stimulate the inflammation and other biological changes that make plaques malignant. They were key contributors to heart disease in the Framingham Heart Study and many studies since, and that's why they're core parts of the ASCVD risk score. Unless you check, you won't know whether your numbers are normal, especially because they don't cause symptoms in the early phases when they're most treatable.

Thus, the most important next step is screening to know these numbers so if they're high you can get help to get them back under control. This way, they don't promote the growth of malignant plaques. What's particularly scary is that over half of the adult population in the United States has elevations in at least one of the Big Three, and many don't know it. They're also becoming more common in kids, which is even scarier. Let's learn more about them one at a time.

Blood Cholesterol

Blood cholesterol is a key promoter of plaque development, but it takes a blood test to know your numbers. Because it's so important, and detection and treatment of elevated levels can provide a normal lifespan, the CDC recommends checking levels starting at age 9.[109] Some countries screen as young as 5 to catch familial hypercholesterolemia. Your blood test will typically give you multiple cholesterol numbers, which can be confusing (explained at FHDLC.info/cholesterol).[110] I try to tell my patients not to focus on the total but on the good and bad cholesterol. Two people can have identical total cholesterol numbers with very different risks. How can that be? Well, if you have high levels of bad cholesterol and low levels of good, you'd be at high risk. But your friend could have the same total cholesterol with high levels of good cholesterol and low levels of bad and have low risk.

Let's start with the bad cholesterol. The main one you'll hear about is LDL, for *low-density lipoprotein*. A lipoprotein, as the name implies, is a particle that's a combination of fats (lipid) and protein, and it carries cholesterol in the blood. LDL strongly correlates with heart disease risk and plaque buildup and is the main target of preventive medications. The ideal LDL level, per the AHA, is below 100 (in mg/dl). While test reports don't flag LDL as being high until 130 or above, I don't consider an LDL of 100–130 "normal." While it may be common in the United States, it's not necessarily healthy. The LDL level we're born with is around 60, which is the same for human societies that still follow a hunter-gatherer lifestyle and have very low risk for heart disease. So, a "normal" LDL on a lab report can be misleading because it can be double those low, super healthy levels. The thing to remember is that the "L" for LDL means you want it Low for heart health.

HDL, for *high-density lipoprotein*, is called good cholesterol because higher levels are associated with less heart disease. The ideal level is above 60 (mg/dl), while the low, most-concerning level is different for men and women—under 50 for women and under 40 for men. The thing to remember is that the "H" for HDL means you want it High for heart health.

The other main part of the cholesterol panel you'll see in your blood test results are the *triglycerides*. This is another way your body carries fat in the bloodstream, and it can go up after meals, like your blood sugar. That's one reason why your health care provider may ask for a fasting cholesterol profile. Triglycerides are also a bad cholesterol, but they only have about a 20% contribution to risk compared to LDL.

A simpler approach to understanding your cholesterol numbers is to look at your "non-HDL" cholesterol. This is simply the total cholesterol minus the HDL. By subtracting the good HDL, the non-HDL cholesterol represents all the bad cholesterol in one value. In some populations, particularly Asians and South Asians whose triglyceride may be more abnormal than their LDL, the non-HDL cholesterol can better reflect risk over just the LDL. The ideal non-HDL level is under 130, with over 160 considered high compared to the average in the United States.

We've also discussed another bad member of the cholesterol "family"—lipoprotein(a), or Lp(a). While Lp(a) is not part of the AS-CVD risk score calculation, it's one of those risk-enhancing factors you may want to talk with your provider about checking, especially if you have a family history of heart disease.

Someday soon, maybe even before this book comes out, the main cholesterol test may simply be the *apolipoprotein B* level (or apoB). That's because all the bad cholesterol lipoproteins, including LDL and Lp(a), have one apoB on their surface, so the apoB level is a better measure of the number of all these bad particles. It's these particles that get into our blood vessel wall and promote plaque growth. So, while non-HDL and apoB are both measurements of bad cholesterol, clinical studies are showing that using the apoB level to measure the actual number of bad cholesterol particles helps provide a more precise indicator of future risk and better identify who will benefit the most from therapy.[111]

My last comment on knowing your cholesterol numbers is that they're just one of the many factors to consider. What is a "healthy" cholesterol level for you may depend on many factors, including your family history and genes and all the other risk factors we've been discussing. If you have concerns, don't let your provider tell you that you can't have heart disease because your cholesterol is normal. I've had too many friends and colleagues tell me that their provider stops after checking cholesterol. There can be many other contributors to plaque buildup that must be considered.

Blood Pressure

High blood pressure, or *hypertension*, has become the most common heart disease and stroke risk factor in the world and the number one cause of global deaths. It's now present in half of the adult population in the United States. As the name indicates, it's the pressure of the blood inside our vessels. Specifically, it's the pressure inside our arteries, including the ones that supply our heart and brain. When the heart pumps, it raises the pressure of the blood so it can supply the rest of the body, just like the water pressure in pipes must start at a high enough level to supply a home. If the pressure in our arteries is too high, however, there's too much stress on our blood vessel wall and that promotes plaque formation and growth. Because this stress and plaque happens in the arteries that supply our heart and brain, that's why high blood pressure can cause heart attacks and strokes.

How do we measure blood pressure? In the hospital, we can insert a catheter directly into a blood vessel, but of course, we'd prefer to take the measurement noninvasively. The traditional way is in the clinic with a cuff and a stethoscope. The cuff goes around the arm and is inflated so the pressure in the cuff is above that in the artery. This compresses the artery and stops blood flow. That's why it can start to hurt if the cuff is left inflated too long. As the air is released from the cuff, the pressure drops to where your blood vessel can open again. Recall that the heartbeat has two phases: *systolic*—when it squeezes and pumps blood out and *diastolic*—when it relaxes and fills up with blood. So, blood pressure goes up in systole and down in diastole. When the cuff pressure is in between the systolic and diastolic blood pressure, the artery can open briefly during each heartbeat. That's what we listen for with the stethoscope—the brief sounds that happen as the artery opens and closes and lets some blood flow through. When those sounds are first heard, that's when the cuff pressure (which you can see on the dial) equals the systolic blood pressure. When the cuff pressure drops enough so the sounds go away, that's the diastolic blood pressure because the artery now stays open all the time. That explains why your blood pressure is given in two numbers, like 110/70, representing both the higher systolic and lower diastolic pressures.

It's now more common to use an automated blood pressure machine, even in clinics. That still uses a cuff that inflates around your arm, but the machine now detects when the cuff pressure is between the systolic and diastolic blood pressure, so no stethoscope is needed. These automated machines are what you'll find freely available to use in many pharmacies, and it's the same technology in machines you can buy for home use.

Because high blood pressure is common and a big risk factor, all adults 18 and over should be screened. The American Academy of

Pediatrics and AHA recommend screening children starting at age 3.[112] Unfortunately, many people don't know they have high blood pressure, even though getting checked in a clinic or pharmacy should be accessible for all. It's important to know that blood pressure can vary with activity, caffeine, and other factors, so it's essential to follow the instructions when doing it yourself. The main thing I see in my practice is that people don't sit for five minutes before checking. I'm not always patient myself, so when I put on the cuff, I read something (hopefully not stress inducing) for five minutes before pressing the start button. I'm a strong believer in home blood pressure checks because when patients come into the clinic, they're often stressed and the staff are often rushed, so the numbers are higher than usual. When the measurements in the clinic are regularly higher than at home, we call that "white coat" hypertension (a lot of clinicians wear white coats). The most important blood pressure readings are what's typical in people's daily lives. So, I ask patients to do what the guidelines recommend, which is to check home blood pressure measurements twice a day (AM and PM) for one week and then take the average for both the systolic and diastolic blood pressures. The AHA has a great video on checking your blood pressure at home (go to FHDLC.info/homeBP).[113]

What's too high? Normal blood pressure numbers are when both the systolic is below 120 mmHg and the diastolic is below 80. If the systolic averages 120 or above but below 130, that's considered elevated, or what we used to call *prehypertension*. If the systolic averages 130 or above *or* the diastolic averages 80 or above, that's hypertension (Stage 1). Stage 2 hypertension is if the systolic averages 140 or above *or* the diastolic averages 90 or above. Hopefully a *hypertensive crisis* will never happen to you, but that's when the systolic is above 180 *or* the diastolic is above 120.[113] You may recall that President Roosevelt had blood pressures at this crisis level, and at the time, this was considered part of normal aging. Thankfully, research has shown how damaging high blood pressure is, whether you're young or old, and we have many effective methods to keep it in a healthy range.

There's been a lot of excitement around developing wearable devices to make blood pressure measurement easier and more continuous than the standard arm cuff devices. The FDA has approved a blood pressure cuff built into a smartwatch.[114] There are also "cuffless" monitors that use artificial intelligence and aim to provide more continuous measurements without inflating a cuff around an artery, but these have had accuracy challenges. More on this later when we talk about the next frontier of digital health. Getting accurate measurements to know where you are, whether in a clinic, a pharmacy, or at home, is the key screening step to get started.

Blood Glucose

The third important number to screen and control if elevated is blood glucose. *Glucose* is the main form of sugar that circulates in your body and provides energy. *Diabetes* is when you have high blood sugar in the form of glucose. The full medical term is *diabetes mellitus*, from words that mean excess urination and sweet. Before they had blood tests, diabetes mellitus was diagnosed by the sweet-tasting frequent urination caused by high blood sugars. Blood glucose, like cholesterol, requires a blood test. While fasting blood glucose is the common initial screen, there's also the *glycosylated hemoglobin* (or A1c) test that may be done. Blood glucose, like blood pressure, goes up and down throughout the day in response to meals, physical activity, and stress. Checking first thing in the morning, before food or exercise, is what we mean by *fasting glucose*. Your body should have good control of your blood glucose then, so if it's elevated (above 100), it means your body can't control it very well. If it's above 125, that's diabetes. If it's between 100 and 125, we call that *prediabetes*.[115]

While fasting blood glucose only tells us the level at the start of the day and for that day only, the A1c test is a measure of the average blood glucose for the past few months. I wish we had the equivalent test for average blood pressure! Normal A1c is less than 5.7, prediabetes is

5.7–6.4, and diabetes is 6.5 or greater. The American Diabetes Association has a helpful guide to all the tests to diagnose diabetes and prediabetes (go to FHDLC.info/glucose).[115] About one-third of the US population has prediabetes, and the CDC estimates that 90% of them don't know it. This is important to screen because there are nondrug programs proven to prevent progression to diabetes. The CDC website has a screening tool to determine when you should get tested (go to FHDLC.info/CDCpreDM).[116]

As with blood pressure devices, there's been a lot of excitement around developing wearable devices to make blood glucose measurement easier and more continuous than the standard finger-stick blood tests. While a smartwatch glucose monitor has yet to be developed, *continuous glucose monitors* (CGMs) continue to improve. CGMs use an adhesive patch with a small, hair-width needle plus sensor that goes just below the skin to measure glucose. This glucose level in the fluid just below the skin correlates well with the glucose level in the blood. This allows people to wear a CGM for a week or more to get continuous readings. Its main use has been to help diabetics adjust their medications to control their glucose. As another emerging area in digital health, CGMs can also give feedback on how diet choices and physical activity affect the rise in blood glucose after a meal.[117] I have patients with prediabetes for whom this real-time, personalized feedback has been helpful. For now, though, knowing your fasting glucose or A1c is the way to start.

Is There a Mammogram for Heart Disease?

At this point, you're probably saying "this has gotten very complicated!" I promised earlier that preventive cardiology is straightforward. Isn't there a simple screening test we can do for heart disease like we have mammograms for breast cancer or colonoscopies for colon cancer? Well, there is and there isn't. Not the most helpful answer. As mentioned,

I've spent most of my clinical and research career at Stanford focused on imaging methods to detect plaque buildup inside the arteries supplying your heart. So where are we?

Well, as you've probably heard, when scientists publish a new finding, it still takes a long time to see how well it works to make people healthier. For heart disease screening, we have the most long-term data for a form of x-ray test used to detect plaque in the heart arteries, developed over 30 years ago. It's called a *coronary artery calcium scan* (CAC), and it uses a CT scanner to detect small amounts of calcium in the heart arteries. I tell my patients it's the "mammogram of the heart."[118] Mammograms detect microcalcification in the breast as an indicator of breast cancer. Normal heart arteries don't have calcium deposits (a normal CAC score is zero), but when plaques build up, they form calcium deposits as they age. So, while the CAC scan can't detect all plaques, because not all have formed calcium deposits, we do know that when calcium is detected, there's plaque buildup. The more calcium, the more plaque and the more risk. This is where we now have a lot of data—the higher your CAC score, the higher your risk for a heart attack.

How Much Coronary Calcium Is Too Much?

Good question! Let's review some numbers. Per public information, many recent US presidents have had CAC scans. Donald Trump has had three, each four to five years apart. His numbers are quite typical, starting with a CAC score of 34 when he was 63 years old and increasing to 133 at age 72. As mentioned earlier, a normal CAC score is 0—no coronary artery calcium detected. At his age, it's common to have some coronary calcium. As we've said before—heart disease is common, but that's even more reason to take it seriously. How would his score of 133 compare to other White men his age?

The National Heart Lung and Blood Institute (NHLBI) supported a large study to learn this—the Multi-Ethnic study of Subclinical Atherosclerosis, or MESA (*subclinical* means that people in the study had not yet had clinical evidence of heart disease). I helped review the original grant proposals from many institutions to perform the MESA study. The data from this study were key to showing CAC scores predict future heart attack and stroke risk in a diverse population. The researchers also created a website where anyone can look up what their CAC score means (go to FHDLC.info/CACscore).[119] If you enter the CAC scores above, you'll get exactly what the news reported at the time: Donald Trump had the typical amount of coronary calcium as White men his age, with about 50% having higher scores and only 15% having a zero score. Even though his score was average, a score over 100 does indicate higher risk and, per the 2019 prevention guidelines, is treated with higher-intensity cholesterol-lowering therapy.[108] We'll dive into treatment in the next chapter.

The Power of Zero

I've had two CAC scans. Why? I'm relying on the "power of zero." I've always been physically active and have taken steps over the years to eat healthier, but my bad cholesterol was creeping up, I was getting older, and I have the genetic risk factor I mentioned—elevated Lp(a), pronounced "L-P-little-A"—that's been shown to increase risk for heart attack. It's a condition that Google helped study, and I talk about it more in a blog post we did (go to FHDLC.info/Lpa).[120] With these increasing risk factors, I was falling into what I described as moderate or intermediate risk. This is a fancy way of saying we don't know whether my risk was still low. I had some good factors—the healthy diet and exercise, plus early heart disease didn't run in my family, but I also had the bad factors I mentioned. So, I decided to do what I do for my patients with intermediate risk—get the CAC scan. This is a way to see how the balance of good and bad factors was combining when it comes to my heart arteries. Thankfully, my CAC score was zero. Long-term data from many studies on CAC scores show a low risk of heart attack over the next five years when your score is zero. I had the second scan five years later and my score was still zero. I'm counting on the power of zero to keep me heart attack free!

One of the important analyses that came out of the MESA study was comparing the CAC scan to other imaging and blood tests for how well it could improve knowing your risk. While the other commonly used tests would improve the risk estimate by only about 10%, at best, a CAC scan more accurately predicted risk in over 50% of those tested![121] That's why, in the guidelines, a CAC scan is recommended for intermediate-risk patients when they don't have other high-risk factors.

What about the Executive Stress Test?

I'm often asked by patients whether they need a stress test. Some clinics offer an "executive physical" with a stress test to screen for heart disease. What is a stress test in the cardiology world? The classic stress test is to have a patient walk on a treadmill and increase the speed and grade (slope) while monitoring for any ECG changes because they could indicate that the heart isn't getting enough blood. Often, it's combined with an imaging test, such as an echocardiogram, to look more directly at how the heart responds to stress. This sounds straightforward, and if "executives" are getting it, why shouldn't everyone?

There are three big reasons I don't recommend this as a screening test for my patients without symptoms. The medical guidelines don't recommend it either. One is that, unlike the CAC scan, a stress test doesn't detect early disease—when preventive therapy is best. Second, stress tests are often normal even when there's plaque buildup, so it can be falsely reassuring. Third, all tests can have false positives, which can lead to more testing and complications. I'll explain.

Remember how we said plaques can build up in the coronary artery wall and become malignant before they narrow the artery? Stress tests don't look directly at the heart artery. They just detect when there's decreased blood flow due to severe narrowing. This means they miss the "tip of the iceberg" we discussed. This means you can have a normal result even with a lot of plaque buildup. This can make the patient, and their doctor, think they're in the clear when they're still at risk for a heart attack. You've likely heard of cases where someone had a normal stress test one day and a heart attack the next. This reinforces what we've been learning—it's about the biology of plaque, so waiting for an abnormal stress test is far too late.

But what's the harm in doing a stress test? We've already said that a negative result doesn't mean there isn't plaque buildup, so that can hurt if it discourages prevention. It could come back abnormal, and wouldn't that be good to know? I wish I could say the answer is yes. The problem is there isn't any proven benefit to a stress test in someone without symptoms, and there can be harm. Stressing the heart to near its maximum has some risk in and of itself. The bigger issue is that, in about one in five people, an abnormal stress test result is a false positive, meaning there isn't a narrowing. Unfortunately, all tests have some false positives—mammograms are a good example. We don't know it's a false positive until we perform a more invasive test, typically the invasive coronary angiogram. So, a false positive means having the risk of the procedure without benefit. I've had many patients come to me for second opinions because their cardiologist may find a partial narrowing and want to put a stent in. The bias of most cardiologists is the *oculodilatory reflex*—to stent (-dilate) any narrowings seen (oculo-) on the angiogram, even when the risk may outweigh the benefit. As you can see, what started as a simple screening test could lead to a false sense of security or risky invasive procedures without clear benefit.

Seeing Heart Disease from Cancer Screening?

One of the reasons I call this chapter "screen like it's cancer" is that cancer screening can see heart disease! Let's start with the mammogram. Recall how I described the CAC scan as a mammogram of your heart—showing similar calcium deposits but in the heart arteries. A mammogram is also a window to heart disease. Like all parts of the body, there are arteries that supply the breast, and they can get calcium deposits like the heart arteries, which a mammogram can see. These breast artery calcifications are not commonly looked for, but one in ten otherwise healthy women have them as well as over half of older women. They indicate an increased risk for heart disease. Because many women and their physicians are more attentive to screening for breast cancer than heart disease, the opportunity to use this information from mammograms should not be overlooked. Heart disease is underdiagnosed in women. This could help many get a signal to assess and prevent their risk because that may turn out to be higher than their breast cancer risk. Unfortunately, mammograms are not routinely reviewed for breast artery calcifications, and there's no well-defined breast artery calcium "score" as there is for CAC. Further collaboration between cancer and heart disease researchers is needed to make this opportunity for enhancing heart disease risk detection in women more available and standardized.[122]

Lung cancer screening is another opportunity to see plaque buildup. Lung cancer is the second most common cancer in both women (after breast cancer) and men (after prostate cancer). However, it's the leading cause of cancer death, killing more Americans than breast, prostate, and colon cancer combined. Years of research have shown that chest CT scanning is a valuable screening test for lung cancer in those at risk, typically current or former cigarette smokers. Because the heart sits between the lungs, these scans can also detect CAC. Studies around the world show that CAC is common in these patients, and higher levels add to their heart disease risk.[123] This is a major opportunity to help flag heart disease risk because the last thing you'd want is to catch and cure an early lung cancer only to die early from heart disease. Not surprisingly, most patients who qualify for lung cancer screening are already at higher risk for heart disease because age and smoking are shared risk factors. Appropriate screening and preventive therapy for heart disease is often overlooked, however, even in those with a smoking history. In one study of lung cancer screening, 98% of patients were found to have risk factors to warrant heart disease preventive therapy, but only 57% were on treatment.[124] This is another cancer screening test where heart disease risk should be considered and where routine reporting and standardization of CAC findings would be beneficial.

Given the marked overlap in risk factors for heart disease and cancer, the detection of either should be a strong reminder to assess the risk for the other. Indeed, there's an opportunity to rethink screening tests to assess for heart disease and cancer at the same time. We just talked about how lung cancer screening CT scans can detect CAC and how CAC scans are also CT scans but with ECG electrodes to freeze heart motion. A combined CT screening protocol could image the full chest for complete lung cancer detection and include ECG to better detect CAC. One study has shown that this combined screening approach would be cost effective. We've talked about how breast cancer screening can detect breast artery calcification but its reporting and grading has not yet been standardized. Beyond that, there's a proposal to develop a combined CT scan for breast cancer and CAC.[125] Given our discussion, a single CT scan for breast cancer, lung cancer, and CAC screening is technically feasible, though much more research would be needed on appropriate use and risk versus benefit. One could argue that we're already close to the "Star Trek" level of technology with whole-body MRI, PET/CT, and PET/MRI scans possible, but we need more research to understand how to use them appropriately.

Eyes as a Window to Heart Disease

One of the interesting aspects of these tests, even when screening for cancer and other diseases, is that blood vessels are often imaged too. An example of this is the screening test for eye disease that can develop in diabetic patients, which involves taking a picture of the back of the eye (retina). Google researchers have developed incredible *artificial intelligence* (AI) capabilities, and recognizing photos is a key one. That's why I can ask Google to find all the photos of my dog Arlie in my photo library. Google researchers studying health applications applied this AI technology to retina photos. They don't "teach" the computer what is a healthy versus a diseased retina. They let the computer "learn"—hence the term *machine learning*. By giving the computer thousands of retina photos, which eye doctors have labeled with how much disease they show, the computer learns the patterns. When you show it a new photo, it knows whether there's diabetic eye disease. With the growing number of diabetics in the world and the limited number of eye doctors, this can broaden the availability of screening and let the eye doctors focus on treating those with advanced disease.[126]

Returning to the heart disease issue, the retina photos also see the blood vessels in the back of the eye. Google colleagues and I studied the question: could these photos also predict heart disease risk factors and even future heart attacks? The answer is yes. The computer learned to "see" age, sex, and blood pressure levels—and for high blood pressure in particular, the spots on the photo the computer was paying the most attention to were the blood vessels. This single photo of the retina could predict a heart attack just as well as the ASCVD risk score calculator.[127] As I wrote in a blog post at the time, the eye was truly a window to the heart (go to FHDLC.info/eyeheart).[128] We'll talk more in a later chapter about the opportunities of AI as well as the challenges of turning research like this into early screening tools that can help you and your doctor.

Key Takeaways: Screening

- Get your ASCVD risk score calculated on your own or by your doctor as the first screen for heart disease risk. Low 10-year risk is under 5%, moderate is 5%–20%, and high is above 20%.
- Know your cholesterol numbers. Ideal LDL is under 100. Normal HDL is over 50 if you're a woman or over 40 if you're a man. Normal triglycerides is under 150.

- Know your blood pressure numbers. Normal is under 120/80, hypertension is over 130/80, and elevated (or prehypertension) is in between.

- Know your glucose numbers. Normal is a fasting glucose under 100 or A1c under 5.7%, diabetes is a fasting glucose over 125 or A1c over 6.4%, and prediabetes is in between.

- The coronary artery calcium (CAC) scan is the main screening test recommended to look for early heart disease when your risk is no longer low.

- Stress testing is not recommended when you don't have heart disease symptoms because it does not detect early disease and is more likely to provide false assurance or a false positive result.

- Early disease in your blood vessels can be detected on other imaging tests you do (such as mammogram, lung CT scan, and retinal photo), so if you've had these ask that they be checked for heart disease risk.

CHAPTER 11

Treat Like It's Cancer

Uplevel Care

Remember when I said I dodged a bullet when my skin cancer was discovered and treated early? The dermatologist was extra careful broaching the "C" word with me, knowing it conveys a fatal disease. Once given that diagnosis, the level of care and consideration goes way up. My sister has spent many years dodging a much bigger bullet—metastatic ovarian cancer—thanks, in large part, to the high level of care and caring at every level—from the nurses, oncologists, surgeons, and imagers to the science and advanced therapies to the family support throughout. This is a model for how we should fight heart disease like cancer—treat it as seriously by raising the level of care and caring to match. As heart disease continues to kill more people than cancer, we're overdue to fight it as seriously.

I should clarify that the treatment I'm talking about here are therapies for *preventing* heart attacks and strokes, the devastating consequences of plaque buildup. Medicine, to its credit, does get serious when people come to the hospital with a heart attack or stroke because rapid interventions to restore blood flow to the heart or brain can be lifesaving. I'm talking about the medications and other therapies we have to prevent the first one because many having a first heart attack don't make it to the hospital in time. For patients who've already had a heart attack, we can provide them with the best treatments to prevent another.

What does it mean to uplevel care? It starts with the understanding that heart disease can be a death sentence, like cancer, if not taken seriously. My father-in-law was a prime example. This means patients, their families, and the health care system all must rethink how we view and treat it. I mentioned early in the book that I was introduced to cancer as an uninformed engineering student. My grandfather had stomach cancer that took him quickly. My first real medical experience with cancer care didn't happen until I was a medical student, where I saw breast cancer patients come to Stanford for "tumor board." A tumor board is a group of clinical specialists who meet to review a patient's case to recommend the best treatment strategy. The medical oncologist would present the patient's history and exam, the radiologist the scans, and the pathologist the tumor findings under the microscope, with specialists in chemotherapy, radiation therapy, and cancer surgery all joining the discussion. This team approach is what we'd all want for our cancer care. Why not also for guiding heart disease care because it's the number one killer? Stanford does have this for complex heart disease patients, where cases are presented to cardiologists, surgeons, and imaging specialists to get expert input. Our Preventive Cardiology Clinic also meets weekly and reviews challenging prevention cases, but this is far from routine in heart disease care.

Another way to uplevel heart disease care is to use all the effective therapies we have to reverse the biology and make it benign. Throughout the book, we've been on a journey of learning how heart disease is more of a biology problem—like cancer—than an engineering problem. The key to treating it is to stop or reverse the growth factors that make plaques become malignant. We've talked about many things you can do—on your own or with your doctor—to prevent heart disease from even getting started. This proactive prevention is based on a healthy lifestyle—the topics we reviewed in the prevention chapter. We've talked about the importance of calculating your risk score and screening for high cholesterol, blood pressure, and blood glucose, so if these risk factors develop, we can catch them earlier when they're most modifiable. We can then use imaging, at the appropriate stage, to help understand if we have early plaque buildup that puts us at higher risk for a heart attack. Ultimately, we may end up where my patient was at the start of the book, with evidence of plaque buildup in the heart arteries. What treatment, or chemotherapy, is recommended next?

As we introduced, the main plaque growth factors are the Big Three: high cholesterol, high blood pressure, and high blood glucose. They also contribute to inflammation, which we'll address. Reducing them are all ways to stop or reverse plaque growth and, most importantly, turn plaques benign. We now have a range of medications to help treat all three. We even have *digital therapeutics* that leverage digital technologies for heart disease care, which we'll discuss in a dedicated chapter.

Reverse the Biology: Cholesterol

Let's start with the main treatment I discuss with my patients at risk, namely the powerful medications developed over the last few decades to dramatically lower cholesterol. We know that cholesterol, particularly the bad cholesterol LDL, is a strong stimulus for plaque growth, inflammation, and heart attacks. Nobel Prize–winning science and decades of clinical studies have shown us the strong link between LDL and dying early from heart disease. Recall that patients with a single genetic mutation that reduces the liver's ability to remove LDL from the bloodstream will suffer heart attacks in their 40s or earlier. If patients have two of these FH genes—one from each parent—they will have heart attacks in childhood and not live into adulthood if untreated. As we'll discuss, there are genetic mutations with the opposite effect, where the LDL receptor works better, and these patients have very low LDL levels and don't get heart disease. Those Nobel Prize winners Brown and Goldstein have reviewed the history of these discoveries in an article aptly titled, "A Century of Cholesterol and Coronaries: From Plaques to Genes to Statins."[129]

While most of us don't have FH, many of us do have LDL levels above the ideal level (100), and far above what we're born with (60). That's why most of us, men and women, will grow plaques in our heart arteries, which we learned from autopsies of soldiers can start in our 20s. As the above article implies, the drugs we call *statins* have been key to our reversal of the impact of cholesterol on plaque buildup because they can lower LDL by 50% or more. Not only do they lower LDL, but imaging has shown that they can turn plaques from malignant to benign. Recall how cancer doctors use PET scans to find tumors, like my sister's, that are active and growing? Cancer chemotherapy can turn those PET scans negative, or benign. Researchers have done similar imaging of plaques to see how they respond to cholesterol-lowering medications. By taking PET scans of plaques in the neck (carotid) arteries before and after starting statin medication, researchers showed that the PET scans improved in a matter of months![130] Statins don't make plaques disappear—they're not a form of Draino to completely clear our pipes—but they do reverse the growth and inflammation that high cholesterol was promoting. Thus, plaques do shrink, become less inflamed, and most importantly they're less likely to burst and cause a heart attack. As we've discussed, having plaques in the heart arteries is not the key issue; it's having malignant plaques—the ones that cause heart attacks and sudden death—that we must reverse. Cholesterol-lowering medications can be considered an essential "chemotherapy" to turn heart disease benign.

With all that's been written about heart disease treatments, including statins, it's natural to ask how sure we are that lowering cholesterol prevents heart disease. After all, many "truths" in medicine are modified when science learns more. The great news is that the latest science and treatments have strengthened the link between lowering cholesterol and preventing heart attacks.

The heroines for the latest science on linking cholesterol and heart disease are Drs. Helen Hobbs, Catherine Boileau, and Sharlayne Tracy. Dr. Hobbs is a professor at University of Texas Southwestern. She learned about cholesterol and genetics in the laboratory of Brown and Gold-stein (the Nobel Prize winners), where she started her research career after completing medical school and residency. Dr. Hobbs wanted to find more genes that could cause abnormal cholesterol levels and heart disease and was able to get funding to establish a Framingham-like study in Dallas. This area was much more ethnically diverse than Framingham, so the Dallas Heart Study enrollment was able to match the Dallas population with 50% Black and 15% Hispanic participants. She then had the idea to look for new genes at the other end of the spectrum. Were there patients with very low LDL? What genetic changes might they have? Would they have low heart disease? Dr. Catherine Boileau is a scientist and geneticist in Paris, France and she had a cohort of patients with FH. While many of her FH patients had their gene mutations identified as affecting the receptor for LDL, she also had patients where the LDL receptor genes were normal, so their FH was unexplained. With Nabil Seidah, she tested for a new gene—PCSK9—and found that it explained the high cholesterol levels in several "undiagnosed" French families. Dr. Hobbs wanted to see if the PCSK9 gene could have a role in causing some people to have very low cholesterol levels. Sharlayne Tracy (not her real name) contributed to the Dallas Heart Study, a 40-year-old Black mother of two, whose story was reported in Nature (go to FHDLC.info/Tracy).[131] While most of us hope to meet the AHA's ideal recommendation of keeping our LDL under 100, Sharlayne Tracy's was only 14. Dr. Hobbs found an association of PCSK9 mutations and low cholesterol in many Black people in the study. Most had levels half of normal. Sharlayne Tracy was particularly special in that she had two PCSK9 mutations—one from each parent, which explained why her LDL was 90% lower than usual. All the other tests she had as part of the study showed that she was super healthy with no heart disease. Indeed, when Dr. Hobbs collaborated with researchers to analyze other ethnically diverse studies that followed people over many years, she found that these PCSK9 mutations were almost 90% protective against developing heart disease.

What was going on in the families and patients that Drs. Hobbs and Boileau had been studying? It still involved the receptor for LDL but in a different way. LDL receptors have to be "recycled"—once they capture LDL from the blood, they bring it into the cell and go back to the cell surface to capture more. PCSK9 is a protein that binds to the LDL receptor and prevents it from being recycled back to the cell surface. The more PCSK9 protein there is, the lower the number of LDL receptors, so not as much LDL is removed from the blood. The FH families that Dr. Boileau discovered had mutations that increased the function of PCSK9, while Dr. Hobbs found patients like Sharlayne Tracy with mutations that decreased it, which allowed more LDL receptors to go back to the surface and remove LDL from the blood—keeping them free from heart disease.

Of course, that's not the end of the story. We're taught that association is not causation—seeing two conditions at the same time doesn't mean one is causing the other. Here we already had lots of data—from Brown and Goldstein and others—that genes that cause high LDL caused heart disease, and drugs to lower LDL, like statins, could prevent it. Now we also had these promising data that genes that caused low LDL appeared to prevent heart disease. Could a drug to mimic this effect benefit everyone born without Sharlayne Tracy's good genes? The answer has been yes! Pharmaceutical companies developed antibody drugs to block the PCSK9 protein. Our bodies make antibodies to fight off infections, but they can also be manufactured. Donald Trump famously received a combination of antibodies that target proteins in the SARS-CoV-2 virus to treat his COVID-19 infection. These antibodies to PCSK9 prevent it from binding to the LDL receptor, allowing more LDL receptors to get recycled up to the surface, removing more LDL from the blood, and so on, resulting in very low LDL—even as low as Sharlayne Tracy's, in some cases.

This discovery—that *PCSK9* mutations can have the opposite effect as in FH—has resulted in a huge benefit to FH patients. Many couldn't get their LDL into a good range with statins alone, so these new PCSK9 inhibitors have been the key added option for them. Even in heart disease patients without FH but who can't get their LDL low enough with statins, this powerful new chemotherapy has great results—not just in lowering cholesterol but reducing heart attacks. There's even promise for people like me with the gene for high Lp(a) because PCSK9 inhibitors—unlike statins—lower Lp(a). These antibody drugs must be injected at home, like insulin, but only once every 2 to 4 weeks. A newer inhibitor works by blocking your liver cells from making PCSK9 in the first place and only needs to be taken twice per year![132]

How low should the LDL target be? The treatment goal is to aim lower when your heart disease risk is higher. The 2019 AHA guidelines recommend "moderate-intensity" cholesterol-lowering therapy for moderate-risk patients to lower LDL at least 30% and high-intensity therapy in high-risk patients to lower it by at least 50%.[108] The 2021 European Society of Cardiology guidelines and 2022 ACC expert consensus, benefiting from more data on the safety and effectiveness of even lower LDL, provide specific LDL targets: under 100 for moderate risk, under 70 for high risk, and under 55 for very high risk.[133,134] This should be shared decision making with your provider to determine your overall risk and optimal therapy.

Reverse the Biology: Blood Pressure

The most common growth factor in heart disease is high blood pressure. We've commented that it was historically viewed as a mechanical problem and a natural part of aging—our blood vessels became more rigid as we aged. What was considered normal for Franklin Roosevelt would now be classified as a hypertensive emergency. Because the threshold for hypertension has been lowered over the years to 130/80, based on research studies, half the US adult population now has hypertension. The good news is that, in most people, it's easy to diagnose and treat, but the bad news is that many don't know they have it, and many who do know aren't treated fully. It's often cited as the most common "silent killer" because it rarely causes symptoms. It's also a common example of complacency because it isn't life threatening in the short term, so neither patients nor their doctors worry about it enough. If we recognize it for what it is—promoting growth of plaques in our arteries that contribute to malignant disease, we (and our doctors) would be more proactive about screening and effective treatment. Even more incentive may be that high blood pressure, beyond promoting plaque growth, directly damages smaller blood vessels in the brain, kidney, and eyes, contributing to dementia, kidney failure, and blindness. Yikes!

How do we treat high blood pressure? Many of the prevention approaches we discussed in chapter 9 have been proven to help lower blood pressure, so that's always the first approach. Physical activity, healthy diet, and weight control all help. So does limiting alcohol use and checking for other contributors, like sleep apnea. Most people with high blood pressure will still need some help from medications. Many blood pressure medications work by reducing the impact of our own hormones on our blood vessels. For example, *beta-blockers* lessen the effect of adrenaline on constricting our blood vessels. Recall that adrenaline is a fight or flight hormone our body produces to deal with stressful situations. Other medications lessen the effect of *angiotensin*—as the name implies, it's a hormone that makes our vessels (angio) tense up. Sometimes a single medication is enough, but in most people, it works best to use a combination of low-dose medications to get the synergy of targeting different mechanisms. The overall goal for most is under 130/80, namely to keep the average systolic pressure under 130 and the average diastolic pressure under 80.

Interestingly, there are procedural approaches to help patients where medications alone are not enough. They also target the hormones mentioned. The carotid arteries have a region that, when stimulated, counteracts the fight or flight hormone system and can lower blood pressure. On the other hand, stimulating nerves in our kidneys, which are involved with angiotensin, increases blood pressure. Here, the procedure is to "denervate" the kidneys to lower blood pressure. These procedures have yet to be uniformly successful, but studies continue to show promise for those with severe forms of high blood pressure.[135]

Reverse the Biology: Glucose

The third growth factor in AHA's Life's Essential 8 is blood glucose. Most people think about glucose in the context of diabetes, when the body can't keep it within a healthy range. The reason glucose is on the AHA's list to control is that the main consequence of diabetes is disease in our blood vessels—from our hearts to our kidneys to our eyes (sound familiar?). Indeed, most people with diabetes die from heart disease. Importantly, even the prediabetes level we discussed increases the risk for heart attacks. If we want to reverse the biology that's making our plaques grow, we must keep glucose under control. For patients with diabetes, the main treatment goal is to keep the A1c below 7%.

As with blood cholesterol and blood pressure, it's often a combination of healthy behaviors and medications that work best for most people with diabetes. Early in my career, there were only a few oral medications to lower blood sugar, and most patients had to rely on insulin injections. Even more frustrating as a cardiologist was that these medications didn't have long-term data proving they reduced heart attacks. The good news for diabetes patients now is that there are many more effective oral medications, with long-term data that they can reduce not only heart attacks but other types of heart disease.

In the earlier stages of diabetes or prediabetes, there's a powerful opportunity to reverse the biological impact on our blood vessels by reversing prediabetes or diabetes itself. I mentioned a patient of mine who was told he may need insulin when he and his wife needed to step in to care for their granddaughter. This powerful motivation helped him revamp his diet and rev up his physical activity. He not only avoided insulin but reversed his numbers and maintained his glucose levels in a good range, even off diabetes medications. More of my patients are now using CGMs to get real-time feedback on how their blood sugar responds to what they eat and how they exercise. This helps get their blood sugar under control or keep from progressing from prediabetes to diabetes. There are also Diabetes Prevention Programs, which started as in-person programs based on NIH research but have become available as virtual or digital health programs. We'll dive into that in the digital health chapter.

There are also a lot of promising technology developments for type 1 diabetics that may start helping all diabetics. One is the so-called artificial or bionic pancreas. Our pancreas usually releases insulin throughout the day in response to our blood glucose level to keep blood sugar in a healthy range. Type 1 diabetics have lost the cells in the pancreas that make insulin, so they need to take over its job and inject themselves with insulin based on their glucose level. With the development of CGMs, they can now track minute-by-minute blood glucose levels. These data can then be provided to an insulin pump so it adjusts the amount of insulin injected based on the glucose level from the CGM. Initially, the data coming from CGMs couldn't be synchronized with insulin pumps, so some patients "hacked" together artificial pancreas systems of their own. I was on a health tech panel at Stanford and was blown away by the story of the young woman sitting next to me. She programmed a small computer that she kept in her purse so it captured the glucose numbers from her CGM, calculated her insulin need, and then relayed those instructions to the insulin pump. It was what allowed her to finally live on her own and was proof—and motivation—for the medical device companies to make these systems work for all.

Reverse the Biology: Inflammation

Early in the book, we highlighted the rediscovery of the important role of inflammation, which is regulated by the immune system, as a potent driver of plaque growth and heart attacks. Statins and other cholesterol-lowering therapies have been shown to reduce plaque inflammation. The question has been whether more specific anti-inflammatory drugs, like those used to treat arthritis and other autoimmune diseases, could add to our chemotherapy options and help further in shutting down plaque inflammation.

Much of the work underpinning the potential for targeting inflammation more directly has come from Paul Ridker. We worked together in the echo lab at the Brigham and it was his idea for the study we did on the effects of daily alcohol on blood biomarkers. He pioneered studies of the inflammation biomarker *C-reactive protein* (CRP). He showed in both the Physicians' Health Study and the Women's Health Study that elevated levels of CRP in the blood predicted higher risk for future heart attacks.[136,137] Importantly, even when LDL was not that elevated, a high CRP indicated increased heart disease risk for both men and women. He then showed that statins not only lowered LDL but also CRP. This led Dr. Ridker to study whether giving statins to those with elevated CRP but normal LDL would reduce their risk for heart attacks. Indeed, that was the result in a study of almost 20,000 patients—those with high CRP and randomly given a statin had half the number of heart attacks or strokes compared to those taking placebo![138] Interestingly, while most patients in the trial had reductions in both LDL and CRP, those who achieved both a low LDL and a low CRP had close to an 80% reduction in heart attacks and strokes. This was showing that to really turn heart disease benign, reversing both cholesterol and inflammation are needed.

At the same time, there was accumulating evidence that patients with diseases that cause ongoing inflammation in the body have more plaque growth and heart disease, including HIV/AIDs and autoimmune diseases like rheumatoid arthritis and psoriasis.[139] Indeed, we looked at this in HIV-positive versus HIV-negative men and found not only more coronary plaque in the HIV-positive men, but that the amount was related to higher blood markers of inflammation.[140] All this evidence led Dr. Ridker and others to consider using therapies originally developed for inflammatory diseases to help prevent heart attacks. *Methotrexate*, for example, has been used for a long time to reduce inflammation in rheumatoid arthritis. Preliminary data suggested that low-dose methotrexate could lower CRP and other markers of inflammation. Unfortunately, the randomized trial of this approach in patients with known heart disease didn't find lowering of inflammatory markers or prevention of future heart attacks. Plus, it had side effects.[141] On the other hand, *colchicine*—a drug commonly used to reduce inflammation in gout, did show that it could help prevent heart attacks.[142] *Canakinumab*, a newer antibody drug approved for treating autoimmune diseases, had been shown to reduce inflammatory markers such as CRP without changing cholesterol levels. When studied in patients with heart disease and elevated CRP who are already taking statins, canakinumab given every three months reduced the risk of heart attack by 15%. This new approach—adding a chemotherapy agent to directly target plaque inflammation, especially in higher-risk patients with elevated blood markers indicating ongoing inflammation—now has growing evidence from large clinical trials. Also encouraging, and further proof that inflammation drives both heart disease and cancer, was that this treatment resulted in fewer lung cancers and lower cancer mortality.[143] More studies are ongoing to confirm the benefit to this anti-inflammatory approach so that it can be added to treatment guidelines and strengthen our ability to reverse the malignant components of heart disease.

Unlocking Our Immune System

A different approach to targeting the immune system that's being studied for heart disease is even more like *cancer immunotherapy*—unlocking the beneficial elements of our immune system to prevent and treat plaque growth. Remember how we said macrophages, the scavenger cells of the immune system, were the "bad guys" in contributing to plaque inflammation, promoting plaque growth, and making plaque prone to rupture, which initiates the heart attack cascade? Macrophages are supposed to be helpful, clearing out foreign invaders and even our own diseased tissue. Recall the "don't eat me" protein that can block macrophages from clearing out dead or dying cells from plaques and how blocking this showed less plaque? Of course, this approach had the usual problem with chemotherapy, because healthy cells could be impacted as the antibody removed their protection, too. We had previously shown that a versatile type of carbon nanoparticle is taken up by macrophages and could be used to kill them with infrared light.[144] Stanford colleagues figured out how to use these nanoparticles as a "Trojan horse" to turn macrophages into helpers, combining them with the "don't eat me" blocker to specifically treat inflamed plaques.[145] They've also obtained promising data by imaging cancer patients getting this "don't eat me" antibody therapy. They showed that this novel cancer chemotherapy reduces plaque inflammation on PET-FDG scans after only nine weeks![146]

Starving Plaques?

Cancer has taught us that angiogenesis is critical for tumor growth—new vessels develop inside tumors to provide the blood supply they need to grow. There's strong evidence that angiogenesis is important for plaque growth as well. The new vessels that form inside plaques not only provide more blood supply, but they make it easier for cells like macrophages to get inside plaques and contribute to inflammation. These new vessels are fragile and contribute to the vulnerability of plaques to rupture and cause heart attacks. Thus, anti-angiogenesis therapies used to starve cancer growth have the potential to starve plaque growth and prevent the formation of malignant plaques. The heart also needs to be able to stimulate blood vessel growth where it needs better blood supply, so angiogenesis is a double-edged sword for heart disease. The initial enthusiasm for growing more blood vessels has not panned out in clinical trials.[147] Similarly, following the cancer lead in blocking angiogenesis has not yet yielded heart disease benefits. With many angiogenesis-blocking drugs approved for cancer, researchers have been able to look at their impact on heart disease. Unfortunately, these drugs, when given throughout the body, have had a range of heart disease side effects (see the section on cardio-oncology for more on this).[148] Our cardiovascular system, both heart and blood vessels, relies on angiogenesis for many purposes throughout life, so it's not surprising that blocking angiogenesis throughout the body would have adverse outcomes. Perhaps, like with the discussion about modifying our immune system, we need to deliver anti-angiogenesis therapy more directly to plaques to avoid negative consequences elsewhere in the body. Molecular imaging colleagues at Washington University have shown promising results with this approach. They used targeted nanoparticles to deliver an anti-angiogenesis drug to rabbit plaques and then showed by MRI that this inhibited plaque angiogenesis, and the beneficial effect could be prolonged with the addition of a statin.[149] This is still a promising yet unfulfilled approach.

Editing Our Genes

Because human biology starts at the gene level—the underlying software code of our cells—there have been many attempts to treat heart disease and cancer by fixing or altering our genetic programming. We talked about genetic mutations that cause FH, which, if untreated, imparts a high risk of early heart disease and death. We've called this the *BRCA* gene equivalent for heart disease. Most FH-causing gene mutations involve the LDL receptor, the receptor on liver cells that removes LDL from the bloodstream. Early attempts at gene therapy involved infecting the liver with a harmless virus that contained the normal LDL receptor gene, with success in animal models but limited success in humans.[150]

The big biotechnology discovery that has revived hope for human gene therapy is the ability to edit our genes precisely. This *CRISPR* technology is what the Nobel committee called "genetic scissors" when awarding the 2020 prize in chemistry to Emmanuelle Charpentier and Jennifer Doudna. When I worked at Verily Life Sciences, we partnered with Verve Therapeutics to combine nanoparticle delivery with their CRISPR gene editing of *PCSK9* to develop protection against heart disease, ideally with a single treatment. Verve has advanced their technology, and based on positive animal data, have started clinical trials. Enabling permanent changes in *PCSK9* genes for the lifelong benefit of low cholesterol and low heart disease seen in people born with these protective mutations—like Sharlayne Tracy—would be great for humanity and put me out of a job![151]

What about Aspirin?

Most of the treatments we've discussed focus on plaque growth and reversing plaque biology to make plaques less prone to rupture and cause a heart attack or stroke. But part of fully treating heart disease is to prevent blood clots from forming on ruptured plaques because that's the key final step in the chain of events that stops blood flow to the heart or brain. Aspirin, for its blood-thinning property, has been a critical component of therapy, both during a heart attack and to prevent a recurrence. For a long time, it's also been used to prevent a first heart attack in high-risk patients. The initial large study to show this was the first report from the Physicians' Health Study in 1989, where over 22,000 physicians were randomized and followed for five years, finding that low-dose aspirin conferred a 44% lower risk of heart attack.[152] But as more studies have been done in broader populations over the last 30-plus years, and treatment of heart disease risk factors has improved, the benefits of aspirin have turned out to be much more modest in people who haven't had a heart attack or stroke. The latest comprehensive analysis of the data was performed by the US Preventive Services Task Force, who recommend (a) a personalized assessment of starting low-dose aspirin in adults 40–59, where evidence indicates a small benefit in those at higher risk and (b) not starting aspirin in adults 60 and older, or stopping aspirin in those 75 and older, because benefits decrease and bleeding risks increase.[153] Note that aspirin is still recommended for patients who've already had a heart attack or stroke, with sometimes alternative or additional blood thinners, so talk with your provider before stopping any medications.

What about Those Blockages?

We've spent a lot of time talking about how prevention, screening, and therapy (as needed) can keep plaques from forming, growing, and causing heart attacks. But until we can work together to help all people get started early, many patients will still first present to their doctors with "late-stage" disease, namely severe narrowings (blockages) in their heart arteries. It's been a mainstay of the plumbing view of cardiology that we need to look for blockages and open them—what's been half-seriously/half-jokingly called the oculodilatory reflex of cardiologists: if you see a blockage, you should dilate it. If it's too complicated to dilate with balloons and stents, ask a cardiac surgeon to do open-heart surgery to attach other arteries or veins to your heart arteries to go around (bypass) the blockages.

As with the careful consideration of surgery versus chemotherapy options for cancer, we should be asking whether these blockages need to be opened or whether chemotherapy is enough. Heart disease researchers have conducted many clinical trials to try to understand the best approach to treat blockages once they've formed. Importantly, opening a blocked heart artery *during* a heart attack can reduce the amount of heart muscle damage, so hospitals have worked hard to shorten "door-to-balloon" time. When it's not an emergency, then medical therapy for blockages can work just as well as putting in stents or doing bypass surgery. How can that be? Two reasons—it's the biology more than the plumbing that causes heart attacks, and opening a blockage (or going around it with bypass surgery) doesn't treat plaque building up elsewhere that can still cause a heart attack.

While writing this book, one of my wife's other uncles developed the classic symptom of a heart artery blockage—chest discomfort when walking. We said that chest discomfort from the heart is called *angina*, so he had exertional angina. Note that we prefer to ask patients about any chest "discomfort" they have rather than only pain. Many describe angina as a heaviness or tightness in the chest rather than a pain. These symptoms are often most notable when the heart speeds up at the start of a walk or when going up stairs or a hill and can then go away when back to a flat surface. One day, he had angina on a walk that didn't go away for a long time, prompting him to get medical attention. Multiple coronary blockages were found on the angiogram. This is a helpful reminder to let your doctor know right away if you ever have these warning symptoms because they can progress to a severe heart attack or worse.

One of the early studies to show the potential of medical therapy in patients with coronary blockages was the Stanford Coronary Risk Intervention Trial, published in 1994 by colleagues I later worked closely with in the Stanford Preventive Cardiology Clinic. Patients were randomized to usual care versus intensive lifestyle plus medical therapy to improve their diet, exercise, and blood cholesterol. Patients in the intensive risk intervention group showed slowing of blockage progression over four years but, more importantly, had almost a 40% reduction in heart-disease hospitalizations. Since then, there have been improvements in stents for opening blockages and in our chemotherapy to prevent heart attacks. So, more research was needed to test this question using state-of-the-art therapies. Fast-forward to 2020 and David Maron, one of the authors of the 1994 Stanford study and now Chief of the Stanford Prevention Research Center, published the ISCHEMIA trial.[154] This study enrolled over 5,000 patients with stable coronary blockages and compared an "invasive" approach (opening blockages) to a "conservative" approach (starting with medical therapy alone). When followed over three years, there were no major differences, with the conclusion that one can start with chemotherapy and reserve the invasive opening approach for patients whose symptoms aren't controlled with medications alone. This is more evidence that changing the biology to keep plaques from growing and causing heart attacks is the best way to turn heart disease benign.

Key Takeaways: Treatment

- Expect your health care provider to take heart disease care as seriously as cancer care. Work together to reverse the biology and turn your heart disease benign.

- Lowering your LDL is the most proven way to reverse plaque growth and prevent heart attacks (and strokes). The higher your risk, the lower your LDL target should be.

- Controlling blood pressure is another critical way to reverse plaque growth, with a standard goal of under 130/80.

- Blood glucose is another important growth factor to keep under control. Prediabetes can be halted or reversed with Diabetes Prevention Programs, and for most diabetics, the A1c target is under 7%.

- Inflammation is a potent driver of plaque growth and there's hope for more anti-inflammatory therapies to help reverse high-risk disease.

- There's promising research, leveraging cancer treatment, on new heart disease therapies, from unlocking our immune system to starving plaque blood supply to editing our genes.

- Low-dose aspirin is recommended after heart attack or stroke to prevent recurrence. Starting low-dose aspirin if you haven't had a heart attack or stroke should mainly be considered if you're 40–59 and at increased risk.

- How to approach coronary blockages should be a shared decision with your provider because medical therapy has been shown to work as well as invasive interventions. Reversing the biology is the key long-term approach!

CHAPTER 12

Treating Cancer and Heart Disease Can Overlap

"Cardio-Oncology"

While this book's theme is how we can improve heart disease care by fighting it like cancer, there are situations where they don't play nicely together. In his book *State of the Heart*, cardiologist Haider Warraich has a chapter dedicated to his experiences, which he appropriately titled "The Morbid Dance of Cancer and Heart Disease."[155] With advances in cancer therapy, this "morbid dance" occurs more often, leading to a new specialty called *cardio-oncology*. While it may sound like a specialty that treats heart disease like cancer, it focuses instead on the heart diseases you can get from cancer treatment. It's become an important part of modern cancer care to have physicians specialized in protecting the heart.

In my early days on the Stanford faculty, I had several clinic patients who'd benefited from radiation therapy to cure their Hodgkin's lymphoma years before. Stanford radiologist Henry Kaplan and oncologist Saul Rosenberg pioneered this therapy in the 1960s, which provided high cure rates for a cancer that had been quite lethal. What we started seeing decades later, and the reason these patients were in my clinic, was that the radiation that killed their cancer had caused injury and eventual scarring of their hearts, from the valves to the arteries. When the scarring got bad enough, it often needed treatment with open-heart surgery. Thankfully, radiation therapy protocols have been modified over the years, so this form of heart disease from cancer therapy is now rare.

Many new types of cancer therapy have been developed since then, including those that leverage the immune system. The 2018 Nobel Prize in Physiology or Medicine went to scientists who developed this cancer immunotherapy, which has provided a new way to treat Hodgkin's lymphoma and malignant melanoma, of great personal interest. We now regularly use heart imaging to track heart function for patients on certain cancer drugs and use heart medications to help prevent heart damage so patients can benefit from these powerful new cancer drugs.

How Cancer Therapies Can Impact the Heart and Vice Versa

The most common issue with cancer chemotherapy drugs is that they can also affect normal cells, including heart muscle cells. If too many heart cells are damaged, the heart can't pump well enough and heart failure ensues (recall our discussion of heart failure). These cancer drugs may either be directly toxic to heart muscle cells or, by ramping up the immune system, promote inflammation of the heart and vessels. Cardio-oncology involves the upleveled multidisciplinary care we discussed, where cardiologists and oncologists collaborate on risk assessment, monitoring, and treatment. The good news is that the medications we use to treat high blood pressure and heart failure have been found to be "cardioprotective" for at-risk patients undergoing chemotherapy. Because statins have anti-inflammatory properties beyond lowering cholesterol, there are promising studies showing that they can also be cardioprotective.

On the flip side, one of the ongoing areas of study is whether treatments for heart disease can prevent cancer. The most widely studied is aspirin, which was initially used for reducing pain, fever, and inflammation. Beyond its anti-inflammatory benefits, it helps prevent blood clots from forming, particularly the kind that form on plaques that tear or rupture. Thus, aspirin has been a mainstay in preventing further heart attacks and strokes. It was noted over the years that people taking aspirin also had fewer cancers, particularly colon cancer. But at this point, the low-dose aspirin used for heart disease does not have enough clinical trial evidence to be used for cancer prevention, per the latest guidance from the US Preventive Services Task Force. Perhaps the more intriguing research is around statins and cancer. As with aspirin, studies looking at patients taking statins have found lower rates of certain cancers. Indeed, based on several large studies, my sister's oncologist recommended she take a statin to lower her risk of ovarian cancer recurrence. Hopefully, this is another beneficial way of thinking about treating heart disease and cancer together.

What Cancer Therapy Can Learn from Heart Disease

A major goal of this book is to learn from how we fight cancer to improve how we fight heart disease. Recognizing the many similarities in the biology means we should take heart disease as seriously as cancer and employ early detection and use heart disease chemotherapy when needed to turn it benign. Importantly, there are several positive aspects to how we approach heart disease that can inform cancer care. The most notable is prevention. The AHA and other groups have done an outstanding job of promoting healthy lifestyle as step number one to preventing, and recovering from, heart disease. Cancer is often viewed as a random occurrence and not as preventable. Given the large overlap of heart disease and cancer risk factors, more efforts should go into cancer prevention, which we'll discuss.

The other lesson is the appreciation that heart disease can be a chronic condition one can still live well with. Most people develop some plaque over their lifetime. The key is to keep it benign so it doesn't cause heart attacks. Even in those who've had one, we know lifestyle and therapy can prevent a recurrence. Because we haven't invented a way to fully "clear out" plaques from our arteries, it's important to know we can live well with them. Cancer care has typically focused on the idea that every cancer cell must be killed or removed, an all-or-nothing approach. While many cancers can be cured this way, we've seen how many formerly lethal cancers can be managed with a chronic care approach. Prostate cancer is a good example and one I use when talking to patients about heart disease. Almost every male will get some amount of prostate cancer with age. So, the issue is not as simple as trying to eradicate prostate cancer given the potential complications of surgery and chemotherapy. It's an issue of who has a more aggressive or malignant form that's likely to cause problems. Sound familiar? My sister's cancer care is another example of how living well with a cancer diagnosis can involve ongoing chemotherapy to keep it at bay, thankfully.

Don't Forget Heart Disease Prevention in Cancer Patients!

A key topic I don't want missed is how the success of cancer care has been associated with less prevention of heart disease. Because heart disease is the number one killer overall, it's not surprising that it's also the number one killer for cancer survivors. And those Big Three risk factors, or growth factors, for heart disease (high cholesterol, blood pressure, blood glucose) are more common in cancer survivors. Yet studies show underscreening and undertreatment for these pillars of heart disease prevention.[156,157] So, while we started this chapter on the "morbid dance" between heart disease and cancer, we see that there are positive opportunities to improve care for both. We've called for treating heart disease like cancer so we can reduce heart disease suffering. We also want to promote good heart disease screening and prevention for cancer patients because we don't want heart disease to prematurely take the lives of those who've survived cancer.

CHAPTER 13

Digital Health and AI to the Rescue?

The opportunities for leveraging mobile and digital health technologies, including AI, for prevention, screening, and treatment are so important that I've dedicated an entire chapter to them. The premise and promise of *digital health* is to combine consumer-friendly smart devices and smart systems to help us stay healthy. In an ideal world, I could sit on your shoulder throughout the day and help you with daily decisions, look over your measurements, and catch any changes to keep you healthy and out of the hospital. I've trained to be good at reviewing symptoms and tests to make diagnoses and guide therapy, but I'm honestly less skilled at being your daily coach. Even harder is the amount of data we can now measure daily, or continuously, so as a human being, I can't keep up with it all and can't necessarily detect early changes in all this Big Data.[158,159] Also, as we progress through clinical research, our care guidelines get more personalized but also more complex and time-consuming for physicians to provide. One study estimates that a primary care provider on their own needs 27 hours per day(!) to provide full, guideline-based preventive and chronic disease care for their panel of patients, which improves substantially in a team-based care model.[160]

The intent of digital health and AI is to provide this team—a doctor, nurse, coach, and data scientist all combined and sitting inside your phone so they're with you every day—and you can turn them off or on as you see fit and choose whether to share with your health care provider or family. The good news is that this type of digital health is starting to happen, though mostly alongside our current health care system. The more people want regular "health" care as opposed to intermittent sick care, the more we can rebalance the health care system, with the goal to prevent getting sick in the first place. Of course, we also need to provide evidence that this is working. That can take time and learning what works, but we're starting to see success.

Self-Driving Health?

While the main goal of this book is to show you the similarities between heart disease and cancer and that approaching heart disease like cancer can make a difference for you and your loved ones, a key question you may have is how to make this happen. In particular, how do we do this at scale? What do I mean by "at scale"? One of the reasons I made the career shift to the health tech industry and mobile health was to leverage the scale that consumer technology has achieved—reaching billions of people around the world. Everyone needs good preventive health. My preventive cardiology clinic and research on multi-million-dollar MRI and PET scanners for heart disease detection couldn't scale to meet the global need. Even writing this book is an attempt to scale—helping people have easy access to the latest knowledge and tools to make and keep their hearts healthy. I've laid out the prevention, screening, and treatment approaches needed, but implementing them for the world's population is a daunting challenge. That's a key reason I moved over to health tech—we've all seen how people engage with their phones and other digital devices every day for everything else, so let's use them to help everyone with health every day. The field of mobile health has expanded to include many more capabilities of our digital information age, so the best term now is *digital health*. Health has been one of the last industries to benefit from our current "information revolution."

Perhaps the self-driving car is the best example of how digital technologies have come together to do magical things. It combines advanced sensors to track the environment and powerful computers and AI to make rapid, real-time predictions and adjustments to navigate safely, all while sending and receiving information from the cloud to continuously learn from its experiences and update its software. The goal is to provide anyone the most experienced, rapid-reflex driver possible who never gets tired or distracted. This is exactly what we'd want for our health—sensors, AI, expertise, and learning to predict problems and navigate us to great health. As I write this, there are more locations in the United States where self-driving cars are helping people get safely from A to B. Can this digital approach to health do the same? The short answer is yes, but like with self-driving cars, it takes a long time to develop and test the technology to make sure it's "safe and effective" (borrowing the FDA's language), and it must meet people's needs around cost, access, equity, and privacy.

Digital Health for Prevention, Screening, and Care

To help advance digital health for heart health, the ACC and the Consumer Technology Association collaborated to create and release a "best practices" guide for the health tech industry.[161] I had the privilege of co-chairing this working group with Dr. Ritu Thamman, combining providers in the cardiovascular care community with experts from the consumer technology industry. It was recognized that digital health technology, including devices and software, can empower both consumers and clinicians and expand opportunities for heart health. Digital health technologies can help with cardiovascular health promotion, disease detection, and care management.

These three goals probably sound familiar—they align with the prevent, screen, and treat guidance I provide above. We need to promote preventive behaviors, screen to detect early disease, and provide the best care and treatment when needed. For proactive prevention, it's all about healthy behaviors—healthy activity, sleep, and what we ingest. Screening is to let us know if risk factors have developed, such as elevated blood pressure, cholesterol, glucose, or weight. This can help us know when to intensify our healthy behaviors and potentially add medication to get our risk factors under control. Screening also lets us look for early signs of heart disease—have our risk factors added up to affect our blood vessels, like plaque buildup that a CAC scan can detect? That helps us know we need to pursue more intensive therapy to keep early disease from turning into a heart attack or stroke. Finally, if a heart attack or stroke were to occur—unfortunately for some the first wake-up call to think about heart health and prevention—we combine our tools of healthy behaviors, careful monitoring, and intense treatment (care management) to prevent another. We fight heart disease like cancer.

How does digital health help? Consider the self-driving car. The key components of digital health are similar—sensors to know what's going on, computers to process and learn from the data, and AI to provide expert-level help, plus a friendly "user interface" to put your health at the center and, if you choose, keep your provider and family in the loop.

Consumer Devices Filled with Sensors

Let's start with sensors. We talked about my summer internship as an engineering student at Medtronic working on sensors inside pacemakers. The pacemaker electrodes detect the electrical activity (ECG) of each heartbeat and stimulate the heart to beat when needed. The addition of a motion sensor allowed it to speed up the heartbeat when the patient was more active. The pacemaker didn't have a full computer inside, like our smartphones do now, and it didn't use AI, but it was a great early example of adding small sensors to make health devices smarter and better for patients. This first activity-sensing pacemaker is now on display in several museums! We now have many more sensors to measure many more health parameters—most through consumer-friendly devices that take measurements from the outside rather than requiring implants. Today's smartwatches from Apple, Samsung, and Google/Fitbit, for example, include multiple sensors to detect motion and heartbeat, with a much more miniaturized and powerful computer with AI analyzing the data. More on the AI later. Some watches include sensors to measure temperature, blood oxygen, perspiration, and blood pressure. Some can even do an ECG. In our guidance document, we highlighted that there are now many wearable devices developed for heart health monitoring, and they go beyond watches. Health sensors have gotten small enough that they can be embedded in ear buds, rings, and clothing![162] Because many more people have smartphones than smartwatches, including digital health sensors in smartphones has helped broaden access and health equity.

How does digital health use these sensors to help heart health? In our guidance document, we provided several successful examples of cardiovascular prevention, screening, and treatment. For prevention, we cited examples of measuring physical activity and heart rate, topics we've touched on here. Wearables and smartphones have not only multiple motion sensors but gyroscopes, altimeters, and GPS to accurately measure the type of activity as well as speed, distance, flights climbed, and so on. This allows more accurate feedback on the amount and intensity of physical activity we're doing toward the weekly prevention goal. Adding heart rate can further personalize this feedback because age and fitness level can change the heart rate zone corresponding to intensity level—Google has Heart Points, Fitbit has Active Zone Minutes, and Apple has Heart Rate Zones. It's nice to see that tech companies have moved beyond step count to make it easier to get device feedback on achieving the international prevention guidelines of 150–300 minutes of moderate to vigorous activity per week. It's even better to see the growing evidence showing that activity trackers help people increase their physical activity, from young healthy subjects to older patients![163]

For screening, our guidance highlighted the examples of high blood pressure and AFib, where early detection can guide lifestyle and potentially medications for preventing heart attacks, strokes, and other clinical events. While we talked about the work that's gone into AFib screening through wearables and other consumer devices, detection of hypertension has remained a much larger global problem. Like plaque buildup in our arteries, high blood pressure can be silent for a long time until it becomes advanced. Earlier, I highlighted the clinic patient I met when he came into the hospital with heart failure—his high blood pressure had been silently overworking his heart until it couldn't squeeze well, and fluid backed up into his lungs so he couldn't breathe. I saw an even more dramatic case as a medical resident in Boston. A patient who had lived most of his life outside the United States came in with a multitude of findings indicating unrecognized and untreated high blood pressure for many years. His aorta had become very enlarged (aneurysm) in multiple places due to the high pressures, which caused him to have difficulty swallowing and a hoarse voice. The aorta had gotten so large that it compressed both his swallowing tube (esophagus) and an important nerve that goes around the aorta to the voice box. Unfortunately, in much of the developing world, high blood pressure continues to increase, with almost 90% of global deaths due to high blood pressure occurring in low- and middle-income countries.[164]

With hypertension as the world's number one contributor to mortality, effective screening is critical. The good news is that standard blood pressure cuffs work well and can be purchased in pharmacies or online. Most pharmacies have a free blood pressure station. Even with this, close to half of people with high blood pressure don't know it. That's why integrating a blood pressure sensor into consumer devices has been a "holy grail" for digital health for some time. (Not surprisingly, the other digital health holy grail is noninvasive glucose sensing to help with diabetes screening and care, with a rumor every year that it'll be in the next Apple Watch.) There's been a lot of progress with wearable blood pressure sensors. Omron was able to integrate a small inflatable cuff into a smartwatch and get the OK from the FDA because it uses the same technology as the standard arm or wrist cuff. The most promising newer technology is analyzing the pulse waveform that smartwatches use for heart rate measurement with AI-based algorithms to estimate blood pressure without directly needing a cuff and a pressure sensor. We highlighted in our guidance that this new approach needs careful validation before it can replace blood pressure cuffs. Another novel approach is to use a pressure sensor but without a cuff. Zhenan Bao is a professor at Stanford who has specialized in making flexible sensors to replicate many of the sensing capabilities of our skin. We collaborated on a project to make a small, flexible, and wireless pressure sensor and showed that, when placed on top of the artery in the wrist, it can transmit the pressure waveform.[165] We patented this technology and Professor Bao and colleagues formed a company to implement this to help noninvasively and wirelessly monitor blood pressure in babies in the intensive care unit. They're also working on a wristband for home use.[166]

Care Management and Digital Therapeutics

What about treatment, or what we called *care management* in our best practices guidance? Note that this wording is helpful because "treatment" often conveys a drug or procedure, while "care" conveys a more holistic approach. And while we've used the self-driving car analogy, the part that's different for digital health is that it's not fully autonomous— you can't take your hands off the wheel yet. Digital health solutions are designed to help you manage the many aspects of your care, from coaching/educating to tracking your numbers to medication reminders to connecting with your health care provider.

The current term that best defines the initial success and large potential of digital health is *digital therapeutics*. A therapeutic is a medical intervention designed to make you healthier. We usually think of a therapeutic as a drug or device. In this case, a digital therapeutic is when the therapy includes a digital program, like a phone app. A simpler way to think of a digital therapeutic is that it does what we've just been talking about. It uses the smart in our smart devices—phones, computers, or wearables—to help us get and stay healthier. It's health care in our pockets. One of the reasons I like the term digital therapeutics is that it clearly indicates an outcome benefit—you wouldn't want to use a therapy, digital or not, that doesn't have evidence it makes you healthier. And just like a drug or medical device, the FDA requires clinical outcome studies to OK a digital therapeutic as safe and effective.

The good news is that the successes of digital therapeutics today strongly relate to heart disease prevention because many have focused on key components of Life's Essential 8—blood pressure and glucose. The breakout example is the digital implementation of the Diabetes Prevention Program (DPP). The NIH supported the large DPP clinical trial 20 years ago to understand the best way to prevent diabetes.[167] They started with patients with an elevated glucose level (prediabetes) at high risk for developing diabetes and randomized them to an intensive lifestyle program (more exercise, better diet, weight loss) versus a diabetes drug (metformin) versus a placebo (a pill that looked like metformin but did not have any active drug in it). Amazingly, the lifestyle intervention reduced the risk of developing diabetes by 58%! This was more effective than the drug, metformin, which lowered the risk by 31%. While this was great news for the people in the trial, the larger benefit was then creating DPP Lifestyle Change programs for everyone else. Omada is one of the first companies that developed digital tools to help implement and scale DPP programs. It's credited with introducing the term digital therapeutics to indicate how digital tools could be used to treat or prevent disease.[168] Indeed, the CDC has now certified these *digital* Diabetes Prevention Programs, which can combine software with human coaches or even use fully virtual coaches powered by AI. A health coach in your pocket is a powerful companion for the daily work to keep your heart healthy!

In our best practices guidance, we also highlighted hypertension management. Beyond measuring for hypertension as the first screening step, getting the blood pressure under control is key to preventing this dangerous growth factor from contributing to plaque buildup and causing heart attacks and strokes. Hypertension care management involves a combination of home blood pressure monitoring, healthy diet, exercise, and, in most cases, blood pressure lowering medications. That's a lot of things to keep track of, so the aim of digital health, especially digital therapeutics, is to help people with all of this. Providing digital tools and coaching on activity, nutrition, and weight, combined with feedback from home blood pressure cuffs and medication reminders, can help people control their blood pressure. There have now been multiple randomized clinical trials of hypertension digital therapeutics, the majority showing benefit in lowering blood pressure and increasing the percentage of patients achieving "control."[169] There are also promising longer-term data on real-world use of digital self-management programs in almost 30,000 patients, where 70%–86% had substantial improvement of blood pressure for up to three years.[170] Regulatory approval of hypertension digital therapeutics has begun, initially outside the United States.[171]

While this helps people *already diagnosed* with hypertension, we don't have certified programs for hypertension *prevention* yet. Interestingly, we use the term prediabetes for above-normal glucose, and the CDC promotes screening for prediabetes and enrolling in DPPs.[116] On the hypertension side, however, prehypertension was removed from the most recent guidelines, which now simply say "elevated" blood pressure when the systolic number is 120–129 mmHg. It raises an interesting question: why is there a strong effort to screen for and address prediabetes but not for prehypertension? There's good evidence that lifestyle efforts reduce the likelihood of progression from prehypertension to hypertension. In the NIH's DPP study, those randomized to the lifestyle intervention arm also had a lower risk of developing hypertension and less need for blood pressure–lowering medications.[172] In the above real-world study that followed patients using a blood pressure self-management program, those who started with prehypertension had a seven-point drop in their blood pressure. I know from my patients that hearing they have prediabetes is often very motivating to make lifestyle changes to avoid getting diabetes. Should we go back to calling the initial sign of abnormal blood pressure prehypertension and call for certified hypertension prevention programs? The data and the important impact of a digital "HPP" would argue yes.

The other important digital therapeutic we highlighted in our guidance was *cardiac rehabilitation* (rehab for short). Cardiac rehab programs combine exercise, education, and support in managing risk factors to help patients after a recent heart event, such as a heart attack, heart failure, or heart surgery. These programs have strong similarities to cancer care, which is typically approached in a holistic way, emphasizing support services for the patient beyond cancer surgery and chemotherapy. Traditional cardiac rehab programs involve going to specific rehab centers to receive education and monitored exercise. Importantly, this has been shown to improve outcomes and quality of life, so much so that Medicare and medical societies view it as a core metric of quality care. Unfortunately, only about one in four eligible patients complete cardiac rehab, mostly for logistical reasons—getting the referral paperwork, arranging transportation, and cost/access. Even a recent patient of mine who had heart surgery at Stanford required multiple phone calls from our office to get their cardiac rehab set up. COVID-19 has helped push cardiac rehab centers to offer some telehealth options, which Dr. Thamman refers to as "tele-cardiac rehab" in her review article.[173] When my mother-in-law needed it during the pandemic, she could do education and exercise sessions over Zoom!

As you can guess, remote monitoring and holistic care are ripe for digital health technologies. A decade ago, two young entrepreneurs—an engineer and a computer scientist—set out from the University of Southern California to tackle this for cardiac rehab.[174] I met with them a few times, and thankfully, they didn't take my advice! I was mostly frustrated with the logistic issues I mentioned, making sure that when patients were discharged, they were connected with a rehab center near them (plus all the required approval paperwork!). They were looking beyond that and saw that the bigger potential was to leverage digital health tools to let people access cardiac rehab remotely. They combined their engineering expertise with a proven Stanford cardiac rehab program to create what is now the number one provider of virtual remote cardiac rehab. Because cardiac rehab involves monitoring multiple heart health parameters from physical activity to heart rate to blood pressure, there's an opportunity to leverage consumer-friendly devices. Indeed, Kaiser partnered with Samsung to implement a virtual cardiac rehab program that combined a wearable and smartphone app. They found that completion rate increased to over 80% with a rehospitalization rate for recurrent heart problems under 2%![175] Both the AHA and ACC now support home-based cardiac rehab to broaden access.[176]

What Is "Artificial" Intelligence and How Can It Help?

Let's talk about AI. It's one of the most important parts of digital health, but it can sound scary because it contains the term *artificial* and is often described as taking over for health decisions. AI stands for artificial intelligence, which means using computers to try to do smart things that we've relied on human intelligence to do. Maybe "computer intelligence" would be a more descriptive term. The early forms of AI were computer programs that gave the computer instructions to do what a human thought it should do in various situations. When I started at MIT, I thought I wanted to study computer science before I became more interested in electrical and biomedical engineering. I took a computer science class my freshman year and it included writing an "AI" program based on one of the first such programs created at MIT in the 1960s—yes, the 1960s. The original program was named ELIZA. It was designed to have the computer ask questions and then respond to people's answers with additional questions—what we now call a chatbot, long before Siri and Alexa. The most famous application of this program was called DOCTOR, ironically, and it was written to emulate a basic question and answer conversation with a psychotherapist. The program wasn't that "artificial" or "intelligent"—it used basic rules programmed by a human (even a college freshman like me)—but it did usher in the idea that computers could do simple things we used to think only humans could do, like conducting a conversation or psychotherapy session. The full story of ELIZA—and how people who used it found it helpful—is super interesting itself. If you want to read more on what happened when the creator of ELIZA had his assistant try it, check out this podcast that goes into the story. It includes how the original MIT computer code was rediscovered by a guy whose dad was a doctor trying to write a program to diagnose heart disease (go to FHDLC .info/ELIZA)![177]

Most people are probably more familiar with AI achieving the big milestones of beating a human expert at board games like chess. IBM's "Deep Blue" beat Gary Kasparov on the second try, in 1997—after a software upgrade, of course. This was still based on humans programming a computer with all the rules of chess, but computers had advanced enough to have the advantage of testing many different moves, much faster than a human. This seemed like the pinnacle of AI—faster versions of humans with bigger memories, and they don't get tired or hungry.

What's so different about AI now? Why did the CEO of Google say in 2018 that AI could become more important "than fire and electricity"? The simple explanation is that we've flipped the model for how we teach computers to solve problems. Instead of giving the computer instructions on how to get the answer based on what humans know, we give the computer many examples of the answer and let it learn the best way to solve the problem. The computer can, thus, "learn" for itself. Famously, scientists at DeepMind (now part of Google) developed a chess-playing program they called AlphaZero because it started from zero knowledge on the best way to win at chess. Thanks to running on an incredibly powerful computer, AlphaZero could play many chess games super fast to get to the answer of winning or losing. It basically played itself repeatedly, starting with uneducated, random moves and learning with each game which ones made winning most likely. In less than a day, it learned so well it could beat the best chess program that existed, which, itself, could beat humans regularly. But what was most exciting, and maybe a bit scary, is that AlphaZero, having learned from scratch, was making chess moves that no one had seen or thought of before. Per one of its creators, it was "no longer constrained by the limits of human knowledge." It's now contributing to human knowledge— grandmaster human chess players are learning new ways to play chess from a computer!

The term for this new era of AI is *machine learning*. Humans help initiate "training" by providing information on the desired answer or outcome. Then the machine (computer) learns to solve the problem from there, often better and faster than we can and with new insights. How do we apply this to heart health? We talked about my work with the team at Google to train a computer with photos of the back of the eye. Through machine learning, it could predict age, gender, blood pressure, glucose, and future risk of heart attack.[128] I'll have an update on that later, but there are many important examples for both heart disease and cancer.

You may recall that my heart disease journey started with the ECG during college, then the echocardiogram during fellowship, and returned full circle when I worked at Google and Fitbit to put an ECG with AI on your wrist. One of the most exciting applications of AI brings these together. Paul Friedman is another engineer-turned-cardiologist I met during medical school together. He's now the chief of cardiology at Mayo Clinic! With all the heart care that Mayo Clinic does, they have a giant database of heart tests, including ECGs and echocardiograms. He knows well that people with poor heart function often don't show up until they get very sick and short of breath and end up in the hospital (just like my heart failure patient described earlier). Because poor heart function is treatable, it would be great to detect it before symptoms develop. Dr. Friedman's team wondered if the information in the ECG, which shows just the electrical activity of the heart, would be enough for a computer to detect poor heart function, which typically requires an echocardiogram to directly visualize the heart muscle contracting. To test the idea, they applied the machine learning AI approach. Namely, they gave the computer almost 100,000 ECGs paired with the echocardiogram report on heart function from the same patient. With half of the ECGs, they let the computer learn to associate them with heart function. Then the computer applied what it learned to the other 50,000 ECGs it hadn't seen. It worked! The computer was correct over 85% of the time in predicting which ECGs were from patients with poor heart function. It even learned something that wasn't planned—even in patients with good heart function on the echo, it could predict from the ECG the patients with a much higher risk of developing poor heart function in the future! This study used the conventional ECG, where they stick electrodes over your chest, arms, and legs. I've asked Dr. Friedman the logical question about testing with the simpler ECGs many people can now do on their smartwatches. He told me it works almost as well and he made a video to show the app they made to contribute ECGs to this study (go to FHDLC.info/Friedman).[178] Importantly, they've taken this AI algorithm a step further and showed that it can help primary care doctors find new patients with poor heart function,[179] so now they're working with several companies to implement this and other algorithms in bedside and smartwatch ECGs, with "breakthrough" designations from the FDA.[180]

In many ways, we're still early in developing AI to help with health care, but it's encouraging that the FDA's 2022 update to its database on approved AI algorithms had grown to over 500. The vast majority are for cardiovascular and radiology applications, putting detection of heart disease and cancer at the top of the list. It's also exciting to see multiple companies implementing some of the dual screening opportunities we've discussed. Recall that mammograms include the arteries that supply the breast, and seeing breast artery calcification could help women know that heart disease has started. But most of the time, the radiologist is focused on whether there's breast cancer and doesn't review or report on the breast artery calcification. Now two companies that already have AI systems to help read mammograms for breast cancer are working on adding AI-guided detection and quantification of breast artery calcification to help assess a woman's heart disease risk.[181,182]

There are many more examples of AI's potential, including the hope that it can give clinicians more time to spend directly caring for their patients, one of the key themes of Eric Topol's book *Deep Medicine* that looks at the future of AI and health.[183] But it's important for me to acknowledge that there are concerns and risks with AI that must be addressed. We've already highlighted unequal access to health and a key concern is whether digital health and AI improve or worsen health equity. Currently, we see examples of both. With most of the world's population having access to a smartphone, this democratization of technology is helping to democratize health care. On the other hand, many early digital health and AI solutions are designed for high-end devices like smartwatches, which present barriers to access. Another key concern with AI is that health algorithms are often trained on datasets from homogeneous rather than diverse populations. This means the AI algorithm may not work on certain racial or ethnic groups and, thus, be prone to missing or giving a wrong diagnosis. The original Framingham risk score had this problem, necessitating the collection of data from broader populations so the current ASCVD risk score can be more accurate for all. For AI, which needs large datasets, there is a similar effort to expand the datasets that go into training algorithms. Thankfully, many research journals, like the *New England Journal of Medicine*, are mandating greater transparency about the diversity of the data and populations studied to promote greater equity.[184]

The last, but not least, area of concern with AI is whether we're ceding control of health care to a machine and taking the clinician out of the loop. This may not make friends among my colleagues, but I think the future we all want will have more "autonomous" AI for many, but not all, aspects of health care, for multiple reasons. One is that clinicians are human. I know from my own experience that when tasked with reading hundreds of ECGs in a day plus reviewing many echocardiograms and cardiac MRI scans (which have hundreds of images each), I'd do a better job if a computer could screen out the normal studies and let me devote more time and expertise to ones with abnormalities. Another is that we're already seeing examples where AI performs better than most clinicians, as AlphaZero did with chess. That should be viewed as a good thing. For example, when Google developed the AI algorithm to detect diabetic eye disease, they realized that they could improve it by training the computer with input from retinal specialists. This meant that the algorithm could provide specialist-level accuracy—this uplevels care for all. The FDA has now approved several autonomous AI algorithms for diabetic eye disease screening, which primary care clinics can implement for broader access. When one of these algorithms was compared to the interpretation of general ophthalmologists, the results would make you choose the computer over the clinician every time—the AI algorithm detected 97% of patients with diabetic eye disease while the general ophthalmologists detected only 21% of those patients.[185] And one more reason is that some AI algorithms can detect abnormalities that even expert clinicians can't see. Like Dr. Friedman's work, the computer can detect patients with poor heart function just from the ECG you can take yourself, while cardiologists need an echocardiogram to see that.

Clearly, as Dr. Topol's book emphasizes, we don't want to take the human caring out of health care, but with analyzing copious or complex data, it makes sense to have humans do what they're good at and computers do what they're good at and, ultimately, give everyone access to expert level care. And just like with self-driving cars, it's a long road to enable autonomous driving, and safety is paramount. Most AI algorithms in health care augment or assist, rather than replace, clinician expertise. And most are for helping with screening and diagnosis, leaving the care to patient-plus-clinician shared decision making.

Early on, I said it would be great if everyone could see a preventive cardiologist on a regular basis to implement everything we've been discussing. But the reality is there aren't enough of them for the world's population, most of whom need help with one or more of Life's Essential 8. Understandably, many people turn to "Dr. Google" to access the latest health information. A cardiologist and former Google colleague, Kapil Parakh, wrote *Searching for Health* to help people get the information they need to navigate their health care journeys.[186] There's also the challenge that, even if there were enough preventive cardiologists, the amount of data we'd need to monitor to keep everyone's health on track would be overwhelming. I'd like to see an AI preventive cardiologist developed so we can provide high-quality heart disease care for all at scale. Recall the ELIZA chatbot? What if that were a preventive cardiologist who could have the initial conversation with you, review your data, and present information to you and your provider with potential next steps on prevention, screening, and treatment? Wouldn't that be great? As I write this book, we're getting closer to this reality. With OpenAI releasing ChatGPT and Google following with Bard, we're seeing much more intelligent conversational assistants.[187] My hope is for these to be implemented responsibly to give everyone easy access to a personal heart health assistant!

CHAPTER 14

The Bigger Picture

Going beyond Individual Effort: From Personalized Health to Public Health

We've talked a lot about what we can do on an individual level, but there's much society should do to help. When I grew up, the controversial public health issue was seat belts. Car accidents were killing many every day and seat belts could save lives, yet making them a requirement was controversial. My dad would always "forget" to put his on, and our job as kids was to remind him—we wanted him to stay alive. I remember one car in which the seat belt was attached to the door, so closing it took care of putting on the belt. That was discontinued because people wanted the freedom to not wear one. A major lesson here was that it takes time to shift public opinion about government imposing health, even for something relatively easy to do. Ultimately, there was a "shifting of the norm"—wearing seat belts eventually went from a government imposition to something that would be crazy not to do. Whenever I read about someone dying in a car crash now, it's often because they're not wearing a seat belt.

The same thing happened with cigarette smoking in the United States. It was popular when I was little, and I remember my dad smoking for a few years. Gradually, there were more rules limiting advertisement, which helped, but it took many other efforts, from public health research showing its harms to treating nicotine addiction as a disease to imposing high taxes on cigarette sales. Ultimately, these efforts helped reach a tipping point where the norm shifted. Smoking not only became "uncool" among most adults, but the less it was around you, the more the smell and exposure to second-hand smoke felt threatening. This resulted in laws banning smoking in public places, workplaces, and so on. It's hard to believe now, but almost half of adults smoked when I was born, and now it's below one in seven.[188] That's been a huge success story in combating both heart disease and cancer. But the policy and cultural shift hasn't happened in much of the world, with over a billion people still smoking every day. Big Tobacco hasn't been fully defeated. It's now using vaping to get teens addicted, with many new health concerns, leading the AHA to call it a health emergency.[95] Thankfully, in 2022, the FDA with a cardiologist as its head advanced its plans to reduce the amount of addictive nicotine in cigarettes to help people quit or not get hooked at all.[189]

Our Food Is Killing Us

The toughest area to shift the norm has been healthy eating. It's obviously not as simple as cigarettes—we know each cigarette you smoke is bad for you. On the other hand, we need calories to live, and not everyone has access to enough calories or healthy food, so it's hard to be similarly judgmental. Still, there's a lot we can do to shift toward a healthier norm. One of my patients had an extreme name for this—"suicide foods"—but it helped him stay healthy. This is the patient who came into the hospital with heart failure after ignoring his high blood pressure for too long. In the hospital, we could treat the urgent problem, but long term, he'd need to rethink his approach. His near-death experience is likely what inspired his new view of food. At a follow-up clinic visit, he said a major goal when he goes to the supermarket is to avoid suicide foods. He recognized that returning to buying processed salty foods could restart the cycle of higher blood pressure and heart failure. He'd reached his own tipping point—his diet and blood pressure had tipped him into heart failure—but that traumatic experience shifted his view to see that food can kill.

I realize trying to call out foods as suicidal or lethal like cigarettes sounds dramatic, but a nutrition expert hosted by Stanford to give a Grand Rounds lecture titled his talk "How Not to Die"—about how healthy food can prevent and reverse many diseases, with heart disease and cancer at the top (video at FHDLC.info/NotDie).[190] We need to encourage as many ways as possible to shift people's views about what they eat. Consider the examples of employees worried about what their colleagues are eating because it raises their health insurance premiums or the Stanford students avoiding meat to reduce deforestation, global warming, drought, and animal cruelty. How can we harness these ideas to help societies and individuals move toward the healthy choice being the routine, not the exception, as we have for seat belts and cigarettes? Just like when I see someone smoking a cigarette or not wearing a seat belt, I have a visceral reaction when I see people eating unhealthy foods. I recall a recent day-long work meeting where we had a team lunch at a nearby restaurant. Not surprisingly, several of the younger employees ordered meat- and carb-loaded dishes. For me, it feels like I'm in a restaurant that allows smoking, and I could swear I get twinges of chest pain from being exposed to this "second-hand smoke." Ironically, my main worry is that they're the ones heading toward chest pain, or worse, and need to be informed about their "cigarette diet."

This is a prime example of how our society doesn't treat heart disease like cancer. In California, companies are required to add cancer warning labels for about 900 chemicals that can contribute to cancer risk. Yet we don't have similar heart disease warning labels. The opportunity is there for labeling foods as risks for heart disease, like for cancer. The ACS, like the AHA, promotes a healthy diet as a key way to reduce cancer risk. Plus, there are data showing that labels matter. A great example is trans fats. Trans fats were found to be a particularly "toxic" form of fat that contributed to heart disease but were a common ingredient in cookies, snacks, and so on. Food manufacturers on their own hadn't revamped their recipes to use alternatives until the food labels changed. Once trans fats became its own required item on food labels, manufacturers jumped on the bandwagon to show zero trans fats. Success there, but so much more to do. This does seem like an area where the heart and cancer societies could do more together. The AHA has a food "approval" program. Could there be foods with double checks for heart disease and cancer prevention? The workplace is another key area to shift the norm. I recall visiting another large tech company for a meeting. There was a wide selection of food choices, but they all had green, yellow, or red labels to nudge employees toward the healthy choices. Maybe they should add what the health insurance premiums would be if everyone ate from the red instead of the green. Google is famous for its food program because it feeds thousands of people for free every day. Many employees eat breakfast, lunch, and dinner there. That becomes a major challenge—access to three unlimited meals per day. There's a similar challenge at schools and universities. Typically, once you pay for a meal plan, it's all you can eat. I'm not sure why people can't see that's a really bad idea. It's asking people to go against their primal instinct to eat, especially when they've paid for it. Behavioral scientists will tell you—you need to make bad choices hard and good choices easy and help people understand that bad choices are killing them.

Equitable Access to Healthy Choices

While a major goal of this book is to help you understand heart disease better and give you tools to help yourself and your loved ones, it's important to recognize that we don't all have access to healthy choices for food, physical activity, or health care. Mia captures well how growing up in a healthy environment was less fun as a kid, but she appreciates it as an adult.

When I was growing up I never wanted to have the playdates hosted at my house because we didn't have good snacks. No doritos, oreos, pop tarts, popsicles (unless they were the natural ones where you could see the chunks of fruit . . . not what a 9 year old wants). Nothing. You could maybe get dried mango on a good week. I would count down the days until my grandparents came into town who, unlike my cardiologist of a father and unwavering mother, couldn't say no to our excessive pleas for ice cream. Over a decade later, I have come to view what I once saw as so unfair, upsetting, and embarrassing as an undeniable privilege. It was a privilege to have fresh strawberries for breakfast, to live near parks I could play at, to complain about broccoli on my dinner plate, to have someone take me to soccer practice. It was a privilege to grow up with access to a healthy lifestyle and diet. Many Americans don't have this privilege to choose to eat and live a healthy life.

A key example is the recognition that there are "food deserts"—areas of our country where people don't have access to affordable, healthy foods.[191] One health care system recognized that this was contributing to the poor health and expensive care of many of their patients. They initiated a Fresh Food Farmacy program to deliver healthy food, which improved patient health and lowered costs.[192] There's been a growing national effort to implement this approach under the banner "Food is Medicine."[193] This, and calls for adding a National Institute of Nutrition to the NIH, emphasizes that nutrition interventions to prevent and treat disease must be viewed and funded like medications and procedures.[194] The AHA, with the Rockefeller Foundation and Kroger, have joined this effort and committed $250 million to build a Food is Medicine Research Initiative.[195]

There are also "physical activity deserts"—neighborhoods where people don't have access to nearby and safe places to be active. To tackle this problem, one of my Stanford colleagues, Abby King, has been empowering community-based citizen science. Dr. King has been a leader in physical activity promotion and population health and co-chaired the 2018 US Physical Activity Guidelines. She was also part of a fascinating study using smartphone physical activity data from 717,000 people across 111 countries.[196] The main finding was that the health of populations was strongly related to "activity inequality." A main driver of this inequality was the walkability of people's communities. More walkable communities increased physical activity, especially for women, and better health.

Citizen science, or science "by the people," involves empowering community residents to collect information about their environment to identify areas of need and collaborate to implement impactful solutions. Dr. King and colleagues have leveraged digital tools in this public health effort, including a Healthy Neighborhood Discovery Tool that lets people use an app on their phone or tablet to map, photograph, and comment on walking routes and barriers to physical activity.[197] Their initiative—"Our Voice: Citizen Science for Health Equity"—is contributing to community-driven public health projects around the United States and the world (videos at FHDLC.info/OurVoice).[198]

Health Equity: Zip Codes, COVID-19, and a "New" Framingham

We discussed how there was a bending of the curve downward for heart disease mortality in the 20th century thanks, in part, to the learnings from the Framingham study and the public health policies that followed. But the 21st century has made it clear that these benefits haven't been evenly distributed. While major declines were seen in the Northeast United States, heart disease mortality remained high in the Southeast. This fostered the recognition that zip code was also a major risk factor for heart disease. Where you live has many social and structural determinants of health beyond the food and physical activity deserts we discussed. We highlighted this in our AHA 2030 Impact Goal publication because the healthy life expectancy is seven years longer in some states than others.[8] COVID-19 exacerbated this health inequity because communities with a higher proportion of heart disease and less access to quality care were disproportionately affected. This led the AHA to step up and champion an urgent 2024 Health Equity Impact Goal, to remove these access and quality care barriers so everyone can enjoy a full, healthy life.[199]

Modernizing and diversifying the way the NIH does heart health research is another important public health approach to addressing health equity. Moving beyond Framingham, the NIH is tackling this through (a) enrolling participants in parts of the United States where heart disease progress has been limited and (b) incorporating digital technologies to broaden access for participation and collect more real-world data. If you recall, a big "aha" moment for me was our MyHeart Counts study, where we consented and enrolled 50,000 participants to contribute heart health research data, all through their phones. A new type of "Framingham" study, called the RURAL study, has been launched by the NIH, enrolling participants in more rural areas of the Southeast to understand their risk factors and barriers to better heart health.[200] This study flips the model for this kind of research compared to the Framingham study and employs "mobile" health research—in multiple ways. First, rather than having study participants come to a testing site, the testing (imaging, blood tests, and so on) was made mobile, so a mobile exam unit comes to participants (check out the video at FHDLC.info /RURAL).[201] Participants are also given a Fitbit to provide physical activity data and a smartphone app to collect other lifestyle and health data, including environmental health factors in the home. It's exciting to see this come together to advance heart health research—through digital health technologies, AI-guided echo, and ultrafast heart CT imaging, as well as the latest in blood biomarker and genetic testing. The visionaries who started community-based heart disease research almost 80 years ago would be impressed with its evolution for the 21st century.

Crashing Planes

Another way health care could reframe the way it looks at heart disease (and cancer) is to approach it like we do a plane crash. Most countries have rigorous programs to review the causes of plane crashes, in large part to learn how to prevent another. If we're saying heart disease is preventable, then when heart attacks or strokes occur, we should look for where the system didn't work as it was supposed to. There are over 600,000 first heart attacks in the United States every year, which would correspond to more than three plane crashes per day! I still think about my father-in-law and what more I could've done to prevent his "crash." Medicine does have this type of self-analysis called *morbidity and mortality* (M&M; disease and death), but the focus is typically on patients who have complications or die unexpectedly in the hospital. Reducing medical errors in the hospital remains a hugely important area to address, but we don't apply that thinking to prevention. We investigate why a patient had life-threatening bleeding after they had a stent placed in their heart artery, but we don't investigate why they had a heart attack in the first place. For plane crashes, each one is investigated to find flaws in the system to prevent future plane crashes. Think of the improvements we could make in heart disease prevention and maybe cancer prevention too if we did this.

I've tried to apply this approach to my practice to make sure I continue to learn and improve. I was recently contacted by one of my middle-aged patients after he had a heart attack at a nearby hospital. I certainly felt like I hadn't done my job as a prevention specialist. I did my own M&M and looked back through the chart and at my note from his last visit. He had several risk factors, and his risk score was in the "intermediate" range. I talked with him about getting a CAC scan, which we agreed on. Unfortunately, he couldn't do the scan when originally scheduled, and he had a heart attack before the rescheduled scan date. Thankfully, he recovered and his heart function has returned to normal with therapy and controlling risk factors. I can't say for sure that getting the CAC scan when originally scheduled would have prevented the heart attack. It would have shown the plaque buildup in his heart arteries, and we would have discussed getting him started on chemotherapy (a cholesterol-lowering drug and potentially aspirin, depending on the CAC score), in addition to further improvements in diet and physical activity. But that may not have been in time. We followed the correct approach during that prior clinic visit, but in many ways, that was still being reactive rather than proactive—we wait until people are seen in clinic to assess their risk. If we want to have time to prevent a plane crash, we need to know earlier—through more proactive prevention.

Apple, Google, and the main *electronic medical record* (EMR) companies Epic and Cerner could implement this—be proactive earlier. In a plane crash, you've probably heard of the "black box"—a flight data recorder designed to survive a plane crash so investigators can review all the sensor data to see what went wrong. Apparently, in a Boeing 787, close to 150,000 parameters are recorded! In many ways, our EMRs contain a similar volume of information, depending on how old we are and how often we've gone to the doctor or hospital. For my patient, while we were trying to be proactive about checking his CAC score before he had a heart attack, we weren't proactive enough. We followed the conventional approach of waiting until he had a clinic appointment, checking his risk score, and scheduling the test. Sometimes patients skip one of their clinic appointments, or they have a more urgent problem, so setting aside time for prevention and risk scores doesn't happen. One thing I didn't do when looking back at this "plane crash" patient was to fully dive into the EMR like it was a black box flight data recorder to see when the first sign of danger occurred. For me, that would have been when his risk score shifted from "low" to "intermediate." That would have been the ideal time to discuss getting the CAC scan and would have been much more likely to change his heart health trajectory to avoid the crash. Why do I say these companies could be doing the same thing? They could write computer programs to do this proactive monitoring of the "flight data recorder" that is our EMR. Unfortunately, they're still mostly reactive systems. I can open the EMR and calculate the risk score, but what if I haven't seen the patient (even via telehealth) in two years, common during the pandemic? Why can't the EMR analyze my patients' parameters once a month to flag me whenever someone shifts into intermediate risk? Even better, let the patient know too. Apple could do this too because they've built a "Health Records" feature that lets those with iPhones aggregate all their health records data, even if it's spread out over multiple EMRs! This *personal health record* (PHR) could be regularly running what we used to call a "chart biopsy"—looking into the chart to find important health issues. Your iPhone could then tell you it's time to have the heart health risk conversation or that you're due for cancer screening (such as mammogram or pap smear), rather than waiting for your next doctor's appointment—assuming you even have one on your calendar. A former Stanford cardiology fellow helped implement something like this at Facebook (now Meta), where typing in "preventive health" would return a list of preventive screenings based on age and sex.[202] This still required active checking, plus it didn't have the rest of your PHR data to make the recommendations more personalized. Google was very early (2006) in helping you store your health records, with the PHR a key product of the original Google Health (version 1.0). While Google has yet to revive that capability for Android phone users, others have stepped in. Dr. Ida Sim was in my Stanford medical school class and did her residency in Boston at Mass General. But while I started my cardiology fellowship, Dr. Sim went back to Stanford to get a PhD in medical informatics—using computers to improve health care. She's since had a highly productive career as a professor at UCSF, combining digital health innovation with primary care practice. We reconnected a few years after she and Deborah Estrin, a computer science professor now at Cornell Tech, cofounded Open mHealth. They saw that mobile/digital health had a bright future, but it needed ways to make sure it would be open and accessible to all. Ironically, at that time, the original Google Health was being phased out. Open mHealth has stepped in multiple times over the past decade to advance mobile/digital health access for all. After I worked with Apple on the launch of ResearchKit—enabling large-scale health research through the iPhone—Open mHealth spearheaded ResearchStack to extend this capability to Android phone users. When I joined Google, one of my long-standing goals was to have them join this effort. My Google UK colleague Alex Trewby and I hosted a Mobile Health Research Technologies workshop that brought Google, Apple, and researchers from academics, nonprofits, and the FDA onto the campus of the new Google Health (version 2.0). (For history buffs, the Google Health campus was adjacent to Xerox's Palo Alto Research Center—famous for where Steve Jobs first saw the mouse that inspired the Apple Macintosh computer.) Shortly thereafter, Dr. Sim published a review on mobile health in the *New England Journal of Medicine* where she not only heralded the advances and opportunities but called for organizations to broaden access.[203] To advance this goal, Open mHealth was a key partner in creating CommonHealth to provide Android phone users with a PHR feature like iPhone users have.[204]

In the meantime, we developed a mobile health research platform at Google—Google Health Studies. The initial studies were on respiratory diseases (including COVID-19) in partnership with Harvard and Boston Children's Hospital and digital well-being in partnership with the University of Oregon.[205] What's exciting beyond Apple and Google providing mobile research tools is that there's been broad growth of this new field of "decentralized clinical trials"—with multiple companies leveraging mobile technologies to enable broader participation in clinical trials by bringing the measurements to the participant over having them travel to research sites. This helps advance health equity and speed up health discoveries because it's easier to enroll a large, broad participant pool quickly and get more frequent, real-world measurements of response to interventions. Furthermore, combining this with a PHR feature means that our phones can be the hub for our research data and health outcomes! It puts you—the user (participant)—at the center, where you can choose which health records to connect to your phone and which to share with research studies, health care providers, family, and friends. My colleague Alex Trewby has long promoted the concept of health data "donation." Can we use these technologies to flip the model around for those most interested—proactively donating our de-identified health data so researchers can make novel discoveries faster?

Bringing this together, we could set up a randomized mobile health study to test the "flight tracker"/"chart biopsy" idea. People could be randomized through their phones to follow standard of care or have the phone check their ASCVD risk score whenever there's new data (age, cholesterol levels, and so on) to let them and their provider know. By following outcomes through the PHR, the trial could generate the evidence to know if it works.

Screen Every Man over 50 and Woman over 60

While the above "high-tech" approach to monitoring heart risk could provide just-in-time screening for early heart disease, we also need low-tech approaches to help as many people as possible. The simplest would be a public health campaign to raise awareness that if you're a man over 50 or a woman over 60, you likely need to be on cholesterol-lowering therapy or have a negative CAC scan. What? Really? I've worked on technology my whole career, so I can appreciate why the heart risk calculation has become more complicated. It allows a more precise and personalized risk assessment, but complex technology can make it harder to tackle big public health problems—like heart disease. When I first learned the guidelines on heart disease prevention, they were much simpler—you could use the fingers on one hand! You simply added up the number of big risk factors—older age (by gender), abnormal cholesterol, hypertension, cigarette smoking, strong family history—and if you had two or more, you were high risk and needed more aggressive therapy. It was easy to check and explain. Then our science got better. We had more long-term and detailed data on who developed heart disease. Crunching the new data generated a better risk-scoring system, but now you need a computer to calculate the number. This 10-year ASCVD risk score, which we reviewed earlier as giving you the likelihood (in percentages) of a heart attack or stroke, is thus harder to calculate and explain. While there are apps and websites to do the calculation, pausing to do this in the middle of a clinic visit can be awkward and time consuming. Most EMRs have a calculator that runs quickly, but it may not be accurate because it uses whatever it finds in the EMR. This could be a higher-than-typical blood pressure because the patient was running late or an older cholesterol value because it doesn't know about a more recent one from an outside lab. I usually pull out my phone to run the score for my patients because I can then make sure the correct data goes in. Initially, I was excited about the availability of apps to run the score and that patients can run these themselves (see FHDLC.info/ASCVDrisk).[107] For most patients, though, tracking down all the numbers that go into it isn't simple. We added calculating the risk score for participants in the MyHeart Counts study, but only a small proportion of participants wanted to, or were able to, provide all the data needed. So, I started thinking about a really low-tech approach. It was inspired by talking to many medical school friends, whom I knew were getting to the age where their risk was shifting to intermediate. I was surprised to hear, even among these physicians, that many hadn't had their heart disease risk checked. I had to explain to them that our risk score keeps going up as we age, so even if you avoid other risk factors and feel healthy, there's a point where heart disease risk has "caught up to us." What is that age point? The ASCVD risk score calculator helps with that because it also provides an optimal risk score based on age, gender, and race.[206] So, I asked the simple question: at what age will my optimal risk cross the intermediate threshold where guidelines recommend checking for risk-enhancing factors (see the "Screen Like It's Cancer" chapter). It turns out this age is 59 for a White male but only 56 for a Black male. A woman's risk hits similar levels about 10 years later, so the threshold age for a Black woman is 66 and 67 for a White woman. Importantly, the risk score calculator doesn't have good data for other races and ethnicities, and it's recognized that the calculator underestimates risk in American Indians,

South Asians, and some Hispanics (such as Puerto Ricans). Indeed, an analysis of future heart disease events in the large UK Biobank study showed that South Asians—making up close to 25% of the global population—had double the risk compared to those of European ancestry.[207] Another study suggests checking at even earlier ages because their analysis found that CAC scanning would pick up early heart disease in 25% of people without risk factors if started at 42 in men and 58 in women![208]

I believe all this makes a strong argument for every man turning 50 or woman turning 60 to have their heart disease risk thoroughly evaluated, if not earlier when they have known risk factors. Cancer has done a much better job of public awareness about when to discuss screening with your provider—mammograms starting at 40 and colonoscopies at 45. Let's do the same for heart disease and promote a simple starting point to discuss getting screened. You can start your own public health campaign—ask yourself, your friends, and your family. Are all the men you know over 50 on preventive therapy for heart disease or have a negative screen (such as a zero CAC score)? How about all the women over 60 you know?

Universal Familial Hypercholesterolemia and *BRCA* Screening

The genetic cause of the heart disease familial hypercholesterolemia (FH) is just as lethal as the *BRCA* gene is for breast and ovarian cancer. The frequency of FH and *BRCA* mutations are similar, too—both appear in about 1 in 300 people in the general population and greater than 1 in 100 for higher-risk populations. There have been calls by both heart disease and cancer specialists for universal screening of FH and *BRCA* because relying on physicians to screen based on family history is not working well, and waiting until someone has the disease before you screen their family is almost, by definition, too late. Plus, we have proven strategies for both conditions to provide a normal lifespan when identified early. We already do universal screening at birth or in childhood for a multitude of much rarer conditions. Why not for leading causes of heart disease and cancer?

There's notable and growing progress on screening for FH outside the United States. Europe began a range of national screening programs starting in the 1990s. Childhood FH screening is now a European Commission Public Health Best Practice because they recognize that "doing nothing is not an option."[209] Their research has shown that, prior to these screening programs, less than 5% of children with FH were being diagnosed, even though therapy is most effective when started early. [210] Universal childhood FH screening is in large pilot programs in many European countries and offered nationwide in two, with Slovenia testing over 90% of 5 year olds every year! The added benefit is that when a child is diagnosed with FH, their adult relatives can also be screened—helping the entire extended family.

The US CDC has included FH screening in its highest "Tier 1" program for "having significant potential for positive impact on public health," so why isn't it happening? It doesn't even require a genetic test because most FH cases can be detected in childhood with a simple cholesterol test. Universal cholesterol testing in childhood has been recommended by the American Academy of Pediatrics and the CDC since 2011, but even five years later, only 20% of kids were being tested.[211] How this simple guideline, which benefits children and their families, is not being followed by most US pediatricians is hard to understand. You can help your own family and friends by asking about every child over 9 you know. Perhaps that would let the United States catch up to Slovenia and make a dent in the 80% of FH patients who don't know they have the disease and aren't on therapy to prevent premature death.

The CDC also has *BRCA* screening to prevent breast and ovarian cancer in its highest Tier 1 program. Unfortunately, the implementation is also limited to screening family members of those already diagnosed. The tennis star Chris Evert was lucky in a way because her ovarian cancer was diagnosed early, thanks to genetic testing she had after her sister died of ovarian cancer. She recognized when interviewed that it was only through her younger sister's death that her cancer was caught—"my sister's death saved my life" (go to FHDLC.info /EvertInterview).[212] That's not how it should be for these devastating diseases we know how to prevent. Remarkably, with the continued drop in the cost of genetic testing, a *BRCA* screening program in Canada is now being offered direct-to-consumer at a low cost to all women and men 18 and over.[213]

Combined Prevention of Heart Disease and Cancer

The public health approach I'd like to conclude with, both as an encouragement for your health and prevention and a call-to-action for the health care community, is to leverage this growing appreciation for the overlap of heart disease and cancer to develop a holistic prevention agenda for both. I've been active with the AHA since I received my first research grant as a medical student and volunteered on numerous grant review committees and task forces. The most recent task force, as I've mentioned, was to develop the AHA's 2030 Impact Goal. To further the AHA's mission—to be a relentless force for a world of longer, healthier lives—we knew we had to promote a more holistic view of health. This also meant recognizing that heart disease is just one element. To really help people with what they care about most—living longer in good health—we needed to think beyond heart disease and recognize that cancer, mental health, and social determinants of health can interact to limit our overall health, well-being, and longevity.[8]

Medicine has typically focused on specific diseases, but that can make it hard for people to know where to start with prevention. Much of screening and prevention is put in the hands of primary care providers, but it can be hard in a brief clinic visit to review all the different prevention steps (recall the study saying it would require them to work 27 hours per day). It likely leaves patients confused and asking—what diseases should I worry about today and what can I really do to prevent them? Reframing the discussion that heart disease and cancer have similar levels of seriousness, intertwined science, and similar likelihood of shortening our health span should encourage combined prevention. The AHA and ACS already both promote healthy living, regular screening, and "chemotherapy" when needed. Can we update AHA's Life's Essential 8 to be for both heart disease and cancer? Should we think of preventive cardiologists also being preventive oncologists and vice versa?

We've talked about how four components—physical activity, healthy diet, healthy weight, and tobacco avoidance—can help prevent heart disease and cancer. The other major shared item is screening based on age, family history, and shared risk factors like diabetes, plus heart disease risk factors of high blood pressure and cholesterol. Screening also includes tests that look for whether heart disease or cancer is present at an early stage, such as CAC scan, mammogram, and colonoscopy.

As you can see, the list of things to do—and remember—can start to get long. As much as I've been a supporter of AHA's shift to promote cardiovascular health with Life's Simple 7 developed in 2010, 7 is still a lot of things to remember to do, and they're not always simple. One could argue that if they were all so simple, I'd be out of a job and wouldn't feel the need to write this book! And while the updated 2022 AHA guidance (Life's Essential 8) has taken out the word *simple*, it's added another factor (sleep) to keep track of. Adding all the screening tests to cover heart disease and cancer makes it even more complicated. I'd propose a combined, streamlined guidance—Life's Key 3: Let's prevent heart disease and cancer together. The healthy behaviors boil down to (a) get your healthy daily cycle of physical activity and sleep, (b) be mindful of what you put in your mouth—food, drink, tobacco, and so on, and (c) get screened when appropriate.

So, this Life's Key 3 simplifies prevention to three core elements while acknowledging that they can be hard for people, and even our health care system, to do. It would be nice to say that technology has all the solutions here—it doesn't yet. But it does have a lot of ways to make Life's Key 3 easier to accomplish. We discussed the 24-hour cycle of physical activity and sleep that our mobile devices can help us track and nudge us to our goals. Unfortunately, monitoring what we put in our mouths is not so simple. More innovation is needed there—perhaps a miniature camera (e.g., a version of Google Glass that's more of a cultural hit)? For screening, we've talked about leveraging our phones to have a prevention specialist in our pockets who can keep track of the screening we need and when, help us understand why it's important, and explain the results and recommendations. Combining responsible AI and conversational interfaces can provide expert-level care that's understandable to all. That's how we could democratize making Life's Key 3 available to everyone and help prevent our top two killers.

CHAPTER 15

My Next (Work)
Chapter

As you've learned by now, my family and career journeys have taught me the importance of approaching heart disease like cancer and driven me to make modern heart disease prevention and care available to all. My next work chapter brings it all together—the imaging, AI, and digital health approaches I've worked on to help us screen for heart disease at its early stages so we can stop it in its tracks. This uses an imaging technology—light—that's super safe, low-cost, portable, and can be performed and interpreted in pharmacies, community health centers, at home, or almost anywhere in the world.

Welcome to the field of *oculomics*—using the eye as a window to our health. I mentioned that one of the projects I helped with at Google a few years ago applied AI to pictures of the back of the eye—the retina—to predict future risk of heart disease. With just these photos, the computer could see changes in the blood vessels and other parts of the retina that predicted heart attacks and strokes. These photos were from specialty eye cameras, but those cameras aren't very different from the high-resolution cameras now part of most smartphones. Also, photos just use light—no radiation from CT or PET scans and no multi-million-dollar MRI scanner. This Google research study was an important discovery, and the publication has been cited by many others as a breakthrough. For it to help people, however, the research needs to be turned into a product that's available to patients and providers. Fortunately, one of my former colleagues from Google's Verily had become CEO at a company that wanted to build upon this research and leverage eye imaging to develop health products to help as many people as possible. I left Google to join the team to help implement this exciting approach to "democratize" early detection and prevention of heart disease.[214]

It may be surprising to hear, but looking in the back of the eye for signs of many different diseases has traditionally been part of the comprehensive physical examination we learn in medical school. Indeed, one of the rites of passage for a new medical student is getting an *ophthalmoscope* (eye scope), along with a *stethoscope* (chest scope), to start filling our "black bag" of medical equipment and supplies. The ophthalmoscope was invented over 150 years ago and ushered in a new era of ophthalmology. There was instant amazement among the early physician adopters that they could use their own eyes to look directly at the arteries, veins, and nerves of their patients—they had found the only place in the body where there's a "window" to this detailed anatomy. Within a few years, physicians doing this bedside exam were starting to see many of the changes we've been talking about in this book. Blockages in arteries, blood clots in veins, and vascular damage due to diabetes were all now visible in the back of the eye—one human eye (the physician's) seeing another human eye (the patient's) to shed light on health and disease.

If all this health information is in the back of the eye, why isn't this looked at by your primary physician when evaluating your health? When's the last time you recall your clinician, other than your optometrist or ophthalmologist, pulling out their ophthalmoscope to look at your retina? Well, I'm just as guilty. While I learned the basics of looking at the retina with my ophthalmoscope, it's not an easy skill and admittedly not one I was able to maintain. I focused more on using my stethoscope and the ultrasound, MRI, and other heart and vessel imaging technologies we've discussed. So, my ophthalmoscope has sat in my old black bag in a closet at home for a long time. Even ophthalmologists, who do this all the time, have learned that changes in the retina are best visualized with more advanced equipment and procedures, so the rest of us in medicine have largely left our ophthalmoscopes to gather dust and ceded retinal imaging to these experts.

I'm certainly an advocate for expert care, but the problem with limiting retinal imaging to eye specialists is that there aren't enough of them to look regularly for the retinal changes indicative of high blood pressure, diabetes, or other damage relating to cardiovascular risk. Indeed, when I recently had coffee with a longtime MIT friend who became an ophthalmologist and described my new job, she said she's seen many patients for eye issues, but became the first doctor to tell them they likely have heart disease and need to get checked out. She can see the narrowed arteries, fat deposits, and more that a primary care doctor usually doesn't. If we could clone her so she could look in everyone's eyes to screen for these changes, we could get more people on preventive therapy. Barring that, we need to find new ways to make this technology more widely available.

What if there were easy-to-use retinal cameras that don't need an ophthalmologist to operate, with AI to analyze the images to provide expert-level readings of any problems? The good news is that there's already exciting progress in doing this for diabetes. The damage to the back of the eye related to diabetes is called *diabetic retinopathy*, and it's one of the leading causes of blindness in the world.[215] Diabetics are supposed to get their eyes screened annually because close to one in three diabetics have retinopathy. Early detection allows better treatment, with 90% prevention of blindness. But in most countries, including the United States, annual screening rates are typically 50% at best and can be even lower in those at high risk for vision loss. Teams I worked with at Google and Verily, as well as others, have not only developed the AI to recognize diabetic retinopathy with the same accuracy as expert ophthalmologists, but they've deployed cameras with AI into community clinics with strong success. They worked with the national screening program in Thailand, testing if cameras plus AI would work well in real-world primary care clinics. They published their results analyzing data from almost 8,000 patients. The AI system was over 90% accurate and matched the accuracy of retinal specialists in detecting which patients had advanced retinopathy and needed referral to an ophthalmologist. The FDA recognized the importance of expanding access to this valuable technology and worked with a company to evaluate their data on 900 diabetic patients at 10 primary care sites. As noted in their announcement, the FDA authorized the breakthrough IDx-DR system as the first to provide "a screening decision without the need for a clinician to also interpret the image or results, which makes it usable by health care providers who may not normally be involved in eye care."[216]

Helping more diabetics get their eyes checked is hugely important, but that focus is for their eye care to prevent their vision from getting worse. Because most diabetics, and even nondiabetics, die from heart disease, we need to use this technology for all it can do to help prevent heart disease and more. When it comes to looking at the back of the eye to detect signs of heart disease, the main thing you likely remember is that most heart disease starts in our blood vessels. While the advanced form involves plaque buildup that can cause heart attacks and strokes, there are many changes to our blood vessels that can occur earlier and, thus, provide warning signs. Some of the early research on seeing changes in the eye blood vessels in patients with heart disease dates to the 1950s and 60s. One of the keynote lectures at the 1964 AHA scientific meeting was on this very topic, how retinal vessels showed evidence of heart disease—almost 60 years ago![217]

What are the vessels we can see in the back of the eye? Like all parts of the body, the eyes have arteries to supply oxygen and nutrients to the cells and veins to remove the carbon dioxide and other metabolic byproducts. For the heart, we said the coronary arteries that supply blood to our heart muscle cells are only one-tenth of an inch. Because the eye is smaller than the heart, the vessels supplying the retina are even smaller—about one-hundredth of an inch—and we call them *microvessels*. While they're super small, they control blood flow more than larger arteries and are prone to many of the same changes seen in the coronary arteries. One of these early changes is impaired ability of arteries to dilate when needed. For the coronaries, we talked about exercise or other forms of stress as triggers for increased work of the heart and, therefore, increased blood flow. Normal coronaries dilate in response. Can you guess what stimulus makes the retina need to work harder and increase blood flow? Light! Yes, stimulating the retina with light normally results in the retinal vessels dilating. Even though these are microvessels, a camera looking at the back of the eye can measure this dilation and, like with coronaries, their dilation is impaired with the Big Three risks of heart disease—high blood pressure, cholesterol, and diabetes.

Now you can start to see how imaging the back of the eye can reveal a lot about heart disease. Because it can see changes in blood vessels associated with important risk factors and conditions, it makes sense that it can predict future heart disease, too. Thankfully, many large population studies have included retinal imaging as one of their initial measures, precisely so they could follow people over time and learn if these photos could predict future disease. One of my former cardiology colleagues at the Brigham, Scott Solomon, oversaw such an analysis on over 10,000 participants followed over 15 years in the Atherosclerosis Risk in Communities (ARIC) study. They did detailed measurements of the retinal vessels and showed that, in those participants who had future heart attacks, strokes, and death, the retinal arteries were narrowed and the veins dilated. They even found that the predicted risk from the retinal image was more powerful than the prediction of the ASCVD risk score we do in the clinic (based on blood tests and blood pressure measurements). Interestingly, the retinal prediction of future heart attacks was more powerful in women than in men. On further analysis, they also showed that vessel changes, particularly enlarged veins, were predictive of future heart failure.[218,219]

One of the challenges of Dr. Solomon's study was the need to make detailed measurements of the arteries and veins from the retinal photos. The development of AI, specifically machine learning, has provided a better approach—give the computer all the retinal photos and let it learn to do it. I described working with the Google AI team to do just this—have the computer, on its own, predict future heart disease risk from the retinal photo, with similar accuracy to the standard risk score that requires blood pressure and cholesterol testing.[127] There are also researchers who've shown that AI can automate these detailed measurements of retinal vessels to help predict risk, which helps to make the predictions more explainable.[220]

The ideal would be for retinal AI to be more predictive than the standard heart disease risk score. That's how I use the CAC scan—to be even more precise in early disease detection and more personalized in risk prediction. After we published the Google study on using retinal images to predict cardiovascular risk, I was asked to review a study that took a novel approach to this challenge. What if retinal photos could be an alternative to CAC scans? While getting a CAC score is not complicated, it does require a big, expensive CT scanner, and it uses x-rays, so there's some radiation exposure. These investigators compiled a large database of patients who had both retinal photos and CAC scans and applied machine learning. By showing the computer thousands of retinal photos and the corresponding CAC score, it learned what in the retina went along with a high versus low CAC. Then they applied the retinal estimate of the CAC score, what they termed "RetiCAC," to datasets that had retinal photos and data on heart attacks and strokes that occurred later, including the UK Biobank study we used. The RetiCAC estimate was not only able to predict higher risk for future heart disease, but it did a better job than the standard clinical risk score. [221] While the study didn't directly compare RetiCAC with the traditional CAC done by CT, the results highlighted that it could be a simpler, nonradiation alternative to help identify those at higher risk and guide initiation of preventive therapy.

While I mentioned the success in training computers to detect diabetic retinopathy, there's a similar condition called *hypertensive retinopathy*.[222] We've highlighted hypertension as the number one risk factor in the world contributing to heart disease and stroke, as well as kidney disease and dementia. It also affects half the adult population in the United States and many other countries. Yet many people don't know they have high blood pressure, and even when they do, it's not adequately controlled. We know that controlling blood pressure saves hearts, brains, and lives. So where does hypertensive retinopathy come in? Recall my MIT friend the ophthalmologist, who said she's often the first doctor to tell a patient they have high blood pressure? The retina can show changes due to high blood pressure, and that can be a more compelling motivator for a patient and their health care provider than an occasional elevated blood pressure measurement. With high blood pressure, the arteries in the retina become narrower and stiffer, with thicker walls. They take on the appearance of copper wires and also become leaky, leading to bleeding into the retina. The phrase "a picture is worth a thousand words" holds quite true here. It's one thing to tell a patient that their blood pressure is above normal. It's a whole other thing to show them that their blood pressure is damaging their blood vessels and eyes—and if that's happening in the eye, then it's happening in the heart, brain, and kidneys. Looking for hypertensive retinopathy has been part of the guidelines for evaluating and treating patients with suspected hypertension, but most primary care providers are not expert enough to do this regularly and reliably. We said we can't clone enough ophthalmologists to do it for everyone. There is, thus, an opportunity to replicate the approach to diabetic retinopathy we described—use AI to help automate the screening for hypertensive retinopathy so any patient and any provider can have access to this important information to guide diagnosis, treatment, and resulting prevention. There's even research that retina photos can predict future hypertension. In a study of 9,000 participants followed in China, those with the narrowest retinal arteries had 17 times the risk of developing hypertension in the next five years![223]

High blood pressure can occur in some women during pregnancy, with a dangerous form called *preeclampsia*, occurring in one in twenty pregnancies and causing one in ten maternal deaths. Preeclampsia is thought to be an immune reaction in late pregnancy that causes multiple problems in blood vessels, particularly the microvessels as seen in the eye, including narrowing (causing high blood pressure) and leaking (causing kidney and other organ damage, plus leg swelling). Looking at the microvessels in the eye during pregnancy can reveal these changes and correlate with how the mother and baby will do. Narrowing of retinal vessels indicates more severe preeclampsia for the mom and lower birth weight for the baby. Retinal changes are more likely in women with preexisting diabetes and high blood pressure, so retinal examination is recommended more frequently in these groups to pick up changes early. Also, once a woman has had preeclampsia, she's more likely to develop cardiovascular disease in the future, and retinal imaging has been proposed to monitor for that.[224]

I mentioned how you can also see nerves in the back of the eye and that seeing changes in the eye's vessels means that the brain's vessels are getting damaged. One of my former Google colleagues helped write a review on *oculomics*—highlighting all the diseases detectable from looking at the eye.[225] After heart disease, the next big area the authors highlighted was *neurodegenerative* diseases, which damage our brain cells (neurons). These diseases mainly manifest as dementia, which many of us have witnessed in older family members. Most people have heard of Alzheimer's, which primarily affects our brain cells. But there's also vascular dementia, where disease of our blood vessels affects the blood supply to our brain cells. Because both nerves and vessels are visible in the retina, it's uniquely positioned to see beginnings of both types of dementia. Of course, more work must be done to detect those signals accurately, but that's the concept of oculomics—many diseases can be studied and detected from this window into a data-rich part of our body.

So can eye imaging detect cancer? If retinal imaging can detect heart disease and its risk factors and there's overlap with heart disease and cancer, you'd be correct to say yes! Of course, the main way that's been true has been to see cancer growing in the eye. While most forms of cancer start elsewhere, a few forms, like the malignant melanoma I had, can start in the eye. There can also be cancer from other parts of the body, like the breast or lung, that spread to the eye, but these are rare. What if the computer could look for patterns in the retina from people who had cancer elsewhere? The most interesting data so far has come from a study looking at predicting age from the retina. There have been many forms of age prediction over the years—analyzing health data to estimate someone's "health age" versus their actual chronological age. In our MyHeart Counts study, we computed a Heart Age based on all the data that goes into the ASCVD risk score. The concept is that bio-markers may tell people and their clinicians if someone is doing well health-wise (younger health age than their actual age) or not doing as well (older health age than actual age) and needs more attention. We learned this concept in medical school because we were taught, when presenting a new patient, to include our visual perception of age. So we'd say, "Ms. Smith is a 53-year-old woman looking older than her stated age." So, what does looking at "retina age" show? At Google, we showed, using AI, that retinal images could predict age well among several risk factors. But another research group looked more closely at the computer-predicted age from the retinal images—what they call "RetiAge"—and how that compared to actual age in predicting future health. They found that a higher RetiAge—your retina looking older than your actual age—was a stronger predictor of 10-year death, not only from heart disease but also cancer. After adjusting for the actual chronological age, high RetiAge was associated with more than doubling of death from heart disease and a 60% increase in cancer death![226] This is more evidence that heart disease and cancer are intertwined and hopefully more in-centive to keep our bodies healthy to prevent both.

One question you may ask at this point is: if all this health informa-tion comes from a camera taking a picture of the eye, what about the cameras most of the world's population carries around with them all the time—the smartphone? Indeed, smartphone cameras have become marvels of technical innovation and have largely relegated our regular photo cameras to the shelf to collect dust (much like my ophthalmo-scope!). While using a smartphone camera "as is" has challenges for getting good pictures of the back of the eye, many attachments to smartphones have been developed to enable retinal imaging, with studies showing good correlation with standard retinal cameras.[227] What's more exciting is that it's getting easier for less experienced health care workers to capture these retinal photos in primary care clinics in min-utes; it's becoming almost as easy as capturing an ECG. Just like what's happened with the ECG, someday soon we'll figure out how to help you take your retinal photo yourself, maybe even with your own smartphone—a "selfie" that would be an amazing way to democratize early screening for all the world!

CHAPTER 16

My Next (Life) Chapter

A lot happens in life while writing a book! We get older, of course, and with that, staying healthy becomes even more of a challenge and priority. I described my own health quandary of having a genetic risk factor for heart disease—a high Lp(a)—but also a zero CAC score. My situation was what one of my colleagues calls a "data-free zone," meaning that we don't have enough data for a specific medical situation to provide clear guidance. How helpful was a zero CAC score in the context of a high Lp(a)? I'd been counting on the "power of zero," but I also knew that zero calcium doesn't mean zero plaque, just that there are no plaques with calcium in them (yet) to be detected by the CT scan. Also, Lp(a) is thought to increase risk for heart attacks beyond forming plaques by promoting blood clots. Thankfully, researchers tackled this "data-free zone" and published a study showing that Lp(a) and coronary calcium contributed independently to risk.[228] I was glad they found that a zero CAC score was still much better, with a high Lp(a) showing a trend toward increased risk (about 30%), while high CAC plus high Lp(a) had a huge increase in risk (about 400%!). After talking with my primary care physician about the study, my turning 60, and having trouble keeping my LDL ideal despite a good diet, we decided it was time to uplevel my prevention and start a statin. I'm happy to report: so far so good, with no side effects from the small daily pill and a nice drop in my LDL. Plus, I managed to complete another triathlon!

On my wife's side of the family, time has caught up to them. My mother-in-law, Lily, had a mild heart attack. As mentioned, she had a ministroke when she was 60 and was found to have plaque buildup back then but had done well for over 20 years on preventive therapy without another event. A few months before the heart attack, she'd stopped her statin without telling me or her primary care doctor. When her next blood test showed that her LDL had almost doubled, it was clear something had changed, so she confessed and got back on the statin. Her LDL came back down by the time she had the heart attack, but it's possible those months off her "chemotherapy" were a contributor. This is a reminder to check with your doctor (please!) before making any important medication changes.

Lily's heart attack was a reminder that we needed to double-check my wife Lena's prevention status. Her cholesterol, blood pressure, and glucose had been ideal on prior tests and she gets at least 10,000 steps (and 30+ "active zone minutes") on her Fitbit every day, better than me! Still, she was getting closer to the age when her mom had the ministroke, and, of course, her father had the fatal heart attack. She then had new blood tests showing a higher LDL. It was clearly time to screen like it's cancer and get her a "heart mammogram." Even though she's younger than I am and most women (not men) her age have a zero CAC score, she wasn't so lucky. Her CAC scan was positive and showed that she had what I introduced at the beginning of the book—"cancer in her coronaries." From the MESA study of CAC scores in a diverse population, she could get a highly personalized result—compared to other women her age of Chinese descent, she was above the 80th percentile! While a high percentile is a good thing for a test score, it's not good for a CAC score—it means you're at the high end, with the guidelines strongly recommending lipid-lowering "chemotherapy" above 75th percentile. She's now joined me in taking a daily statin. While this was not a happy result, we're thankful to know now rather than find out with a stroke like her mom or a heart attack like her dad. We both want to be around for Kelly and Mia and their lives, careers, and families in the years to come. We're also counting on them and their generation to bring advances in health and technology together to accelerate prevention for all.

Another important life development, beyond my day job, has been joining the board of directors for the National Fitness Foundation (NFF) to promote physical activity and health in the United States especially for school-aged kids.[229] The NFF was set up by congress as a nonprofit organization to support initiatives of the President's Council on Sports, Fitness & Nutrition. It was an honor to be appointed to the NFF to contribute my expertise in health technology, physical activity promotion, and prevention. I'm also joining a world my sisters have contributed to for much of their careers because they've worked with communities through governmental and nonprofit organizations to support physical activity and health, particularly among youth. A major initiative of the NFF has been supporting the Presidential Youth Fitness Program (PYFP) to promote physical activity in schools to help students adopt and maintain an active lifestyle.[230] COVID-19 had a major impact on school-based physical activity, exacerbating the decline in access to physical education and sports in school. The 2022 report card from the Physical Activity Alliance gave schools a D–, meaning that three of four kids weren't being helped.[231] We talked about physical activity deserts with schools being a place where we'd hope all kids would have access, but even schools have contributed to a "physical activity divide" based on income.[232] That's why the 2023 national challenge toward building healthier communities includes "Support Physical Activity for All" as a top goal. The NFF's forward-looking strategy to meet this challenge is to work with stakeholders to provide all schools and kids with free access to physical activity and fitness programs by 2028, when the United States will host the Olympic and Paralympic Games in Los Angeles. With the growing recognition that physical activity, nutrition, and mental health can all be part of a virtuous cycle, we have an important opportunity to support healthier students and a healthier nation.

Conclusion

COVID-19 devastated many lives and reshaped our world, but it should also serve as a stark reminder that it pales in comparison to the ongoing toll from heart disease and cancer. As we look forward, we can reshape our approach to health. Our AHA 2030 Impact Goal publication came out in late January 2020, shortly after the first case of COVID-19 was diagnosed in the United States. Presciently, it concluded by saying "now is the moment" to "work collectively" toward a broader goal than just heart disease and "design with intention for what the future may bring." As humanity works to move past this devastating communicable disease, we're still faced with the top two noncommunicable diseases—heart disease and cancer—that deprive much of the world of long, healthy lives. It's time for all to understand how heart disease and cancer have shared risk factors and intertwined biology, and they need equal attention to prevention, screening, and care. Now is the moment to tackle them collectively, to amplify and simplify prevention, and to bring together the best of science, technology, and humane care to provide us all with more years to play, work, love, and live with those we hold dear.

Acknowledgments

There are so many patients, family, friends, and colleagues who have contributed, in ways large and small, to the journey of writing this book over the years. I am most indebted to my patients, who have allowed me to be part of their lives and have provided me with the opportunity to share their stories to inspire others. My family has also helped in myriad ways—from my daughters Mia and Kelly for providing heartfelt thoughts in their own words, to my sisters for sharing their cancer journeys, and to my wife, Lena, for offering her insights and having her side of the family share their battles with heart disease. Robin Coleman at Johns Hopkins University Press has given me invaluable editorial advice, particularly by encouraging me to share my personal and professional stories to help communicate this important topic that impacts us all.

Finally, I've tried to incorporate all the education and inspiration that I've received from countless colleagues, fellows, and students with whom I've had the honor to work as part of the "heart health" science, innovation, and public health communities. This book could not have been written without all this help and encouragement and the hope that we can all fight together for a healthier world.

References

1. Wu JT, Bray PF. Letter: Monitoring cancer with plasma carcinoembryonic antigen. *N Engl J Med*. 1974;290:1439.
2. Tawakol A, Omland T, Gerhard M, Wu JT, Creager MA. Hyperhomocyst(e)-inemia is associated with impaired endothelium-dependent vasodilation in humans. *Circulation*. 1997;95(5):1119–1121.
3. Wu LL, Wu JT. Hyperhomocysteinemia is a risk factor for cancer and a new potential tumor marker. *Clin Chim Acta*. 2002;322(1–2):21–28.
4. Wu JT, Wu LL. Linking inflammation and atherogenesis: soluble markers identified for the detection of risk factors and for early risk assessment. *Clin Chim Acta*. 2006;366(1–2):74–80.
5. World Health Organization. WHO Coronavirus (COVID-19) dashboard. Updated June 7, 2023. Accessed July 12, 2023. https://covid19.who.int/
6. Tsao CW, Aday AW, Almarzooq ZI, et al. American Heart Association Council on Epidemiology and Prevention Statistics Committee and Stroke Statistics Subcommittee. Heart Disease and Stroke Statistics—2023 Update: A Report From the American Heart Association. *Circulation*. 2023 Feb 21;147(8):e93-e6217.
7. World Health Organization. Cancer. Published February 3, 2022. Accessed July 12, 2023. https://www.who.int/news-room/fact-sheets/detail/cancer
8. Angell SY, McConnell MV, Anderson CAM, et al. The American Heart Association 2030 impact goal: a presidential advisory from the American Heart Association. *Circulation*. 2020;141:e120–e138.
9. Centers for Disease Control and Prevention. Achievements in public health, 1900–1999: control of infectious diseases. Published July 30, 1999. Accessed July 12, 2023. https://www.cdc.gov/mmwr/preview/mmwrhtml/mm4829a1.htm
10. Kannel WB. Bishop lecture. Contribution of the Framingham Study to preventive cardiology. *J Am Coll Cardiol*. 1990;15(1):206–211.

11. Mahmood SS, Levy D, Vasan RS, Wang TJ. The Framingham Heart Study and the epidemiology of cardiovascular disease: a historical perspective. *Lancet*. 2014;383(9921):999–1008.

12. Goff DC, Khan SS, Lloyd-Jones D, et al. Bending the curve in cardiovascular disease mortality: Bethesda + 40 and beyond. *Circulation*. 2021;143(8): 837–851.

13. Bundy JD, Zhu Z, Ning H, et al. Estimated impact of achieving optimal cardiovascular health among US adults on cardiovascular disease events. *J Am Heart Assoc*. 2021;10(7):e019681.

14. Canto JG, Kiefe CI. Age-specific analyses of breast cancer versus heart disease mortality in women. *Am J Cardiol*. 2014;113(2):410–411.

15. Lloyd-Jones DM, Larson MG, Beiser A, Levy D. Lifetime risk of developing coronary heart disease. *Lancet*. 1999;353(9156):89–92.

16. American Cancer Society. Colorectal cancer statistics. Updated January 13, 2023. Accessed July 12, 2023. https://www.cancer.org/cancer/colon-rectal -cancer/about/key-statistics.html

17. Cory J. About New York retiring from the "Irish Mafia." *New York Times*. November 30, 1973:32. Accessed July 12, 2023. https://www.nytimes.com /1973/11/30/archives/about-new-york-retiring-from-the-irish-mafia .html

18. Shem S. *The House of God: A Novel*. R. Marek Publishers; 1978.

19. Haskell R. Serena Williams on motherhood, marriage, and making her comeback. *Vogue*. January 10, 2018. Accessed July 12, 2023. https://www .vogue.com/article/serena-williams-vogue-cover-interview-february -2018

20. McConnell MV, Solomon SD, Rayan ME, Come PC, Goldhaber SZ, Lee RT. Regional right ventricular dysfunction detected by echocardiography in acute pulmonary embolism. *Am J Cardiol*. 1996;78(4):469–473.

21. Goldhaber SZ. Pulmonary embolism. *N Engl J Med*. 1998;339(2):93–104.

22. McConnell MV, Ganz P, Selwyn AP, Li W, Edelman RR, Manning WJ. Identification of anomalous coronary arteries and their anatomic course by magnetic resonance coronary angiography. *Circulation*. 1995;92(11): 3158–3162.

23. Schiavone M, Gobbi C, Gasperetti A, Zuffi A, Forleo GB. Congenital coronary artery anomalies and sudden cardiac death. *Pediatr Cardiol*. 2021;42(8): 1676–1687.

24. Heidary S, McConnell MV. Coronary anomalies. In: Kramer CM, Hundley WG, eds. *Atlas of Cardiovascular Magnetic Resonance Imaging: An Imaging Companion to Braunwald's Heart Disease*. Saunders/Elsevier; 2010: 314–323.

25. Danias PG, McConnell MV, Khasgiwala VC, Chuang ML, Edelman RR, Manning WJ. Prospective navigator correction of image position for coronary MR angiography. *Radiology*. 1997;203(3):733–736.

26. Ross JS, Stagliano NE, Donovan MJ, Breitbart RE, Ginsburg GS. Atherosclerosis: a cancer of the blood vessels? *Pathology Patterns Reviews*. 2001; 116:S97–S107.

27. Virchow RLK, Chance F. *Cellular Pathology as Based upon Physiological and Pathological Histology. Twenty Lectures Delivered in the Pathological Institute of Berlin during the Months of February, March and April, 1858.* Creative Media Partners, LLC; 2018.

28. Glagov S, Weisenberg E, Zarins CK, Stankunavicius R, Kolettis GJ. Compensatory enlargement of human atherosclerotic coronary arteries. *N Engl J Med*. 1987;316(22):1371–1375.

29. Libby P. Inflammation in atherosclerosis. *Arterioscler Thromb Vasc Biol*. 2012;32(9):2045–2051.

30. Little WC, Constantinescu M, Applegate RJ, et al. Can coronary angiography predict the site of a subsequent myocardial infarction in patients with mild-to-moderate coronary artery disease? *Circulation*. 1988;78(5):1157–1166.

31. Yock PG, Linker DT, Angelsen BA. Two-dimensional intravascular ultrasound: technical development and initial clinical experience. *J Am Soc Echocardiogr*. 1989;2(4):296–304.

32. Stanford Byers Center for Biodesign. Timeline & history. Accessed July 12, 2023. https://biodesign.stanford.edu/about-us/timeline.html

33. Fayad ZA, Fuster V, Fallon JT, et al. Noninvasive in vivo human coronary artery lumen and wall imaging using black-blood magnetic resonance imaging. *Circulation*. 2000 Aug 1;102(5):506–510.

34. Terashima M, Nguyen PK, Rubin GD, et al. Right coronary wall CMR in the older asymptomatic advance cohort: positive remodeling and associations with type 2 diabetes and coronary calcium. *J Cardiovasc Magn Reson*. 2010;12(1):75.

35. McConnell MV, Aikawa M, Maier SE, Ganz P, Libby P, Lee RT. MRI of rabbit atherosclerosis in response to dietary cholesterol lowering. *Arterioscler Thromb Vasc Biol*. 1999;19(8):1956–1959.

36. McConnell MV. Imaging techniques to predict cardiovascular risk. *Curr Cardiol Rep*. 2000;2(4): 300–307.

37. Goldberg N. *Women are Not Small Men: Life-saving Strategies for Preventing and Healing Heart Disease in Women*. Ballantine Books; 2002.

38. American Heart Association. Common myths about heart disease. Accessed July 12, 2023. https://www.goredforwomen.org/en/about-heart-disease-in-women/facts/common-myths-about-heart-disease

39. Lin S, Tremmel JA, Yamada R, et al. A novel stress echocardiography pattern for myocardial bridge with invasive structural and hemodynamic correlation. *J Am Heart Assoc.* 2013;2(2):e000097.

40. American Stroke Association. Stroke symptoms. Accessed July 12, 2023. https://www.stroke.org/en/about-stroke/stroke-symptoms

41. Gorelick PB, Furie KL, Iadecola C, et al. Defining optimal brain health in adults: a presidential advisory from the American Heart Association/American Stroke Association. *Stroke.* 2017;48: e284–e303.

42. Stanford Byers Center for Biodesign. Diagnosing suspected arrhythmias: an interview with Uday Kumar of iRhythm. Accessed July 12, 2023. https://biodesign.stanford.edu/our-impact/technologies/irhythm.html

43. McConnell MV. Verily Study Watch receives FDA 510(k) clearance for ECG. Published January 18, 2019. Accessed July 12, 2023. https://blog.verily.com/2019/01/verily-study-watch-receives-fda-510k.html

44. Lubitz SA, Faranesh AZ, Selvaggi C, et al. Detection of atrial fibrillation in a large population using wearable devices: the Fitbit Heart Study. *Circulation.* 2022;146(19):1415–1424.

45. McConnell MV, Turakhia MP, Harrington RA, King AC, Ashley EA. Mobile health advances in physical activity, fitness, and atrial fibrillation: moving hearts. *J Am Coll Cardiol.* 2018;71(23):2691–2701.

46. Jauhar S. *Heart: A History; Shortlisted for the Wellcome Book Prize 2019.* Simon and Schuster; 2018.

47. Kitagawa T, Kosuge H, Uchida M, et al. RGD targeting of human ferritin iron oxide nanoparticles enhances in vivo MRI of vascular inflammation and angiogenesis in experimental carotid disease and abdominal aortic aneurysm. *J Magn Reson Imaging.* 2017;45(4):1144–1153.

48. Maegdefessel L, Spin JM, Raaz U, et al. miR-24 limits aortic vascular inflammation and murine abdominal aneurysm development. *Nat Commun.* 2014;5:5214.

49. Medicare.gov. Abdominal aortic aneurysm screenings. Accessed July 12, 2023. https://www.medicare.gov/coverage/abdominal-aortic-aneurysm-screenings

50. Koene RJ, Prizment AE, Blaes A, Konety SH. Shared risk factors in cardiovascular disease and cancer. *Circulation.* 2016;133:1104–1114.

51. Vincent L, Leedy D, Masri SC, Cheng RK. Cardiovascular disease and cancer: is there increasing overlap? *Curr Oncol Rep.* 2019;21(6):47.

52. Narayan V, Thompson EW, Demissei B, Ho JE, Januzzi JL Jr, Ky B. Mechanistic biomarkers informative of both cancer and cardiovascular disease: JACC state-of-the-art review. *J Am Coll Cardiol.* 2020;75(21):2726–2737.

53. Singh J, Blaes A. Shared modifiable risk factors between cancer and CVD. American College of Cardiology. Published April 26, 2017. Accessed July 13, 2023. https://www.acc.org/latest-in-cardiology/articles/2017/04/26/08/01/shared-modifiable-risk-factors-between-cancer-and-cvd

54. Physical Activity Guidelines Advisory Committee. Part F. Chapter 4. Cancer prevention. In: *2018 Physical Activity Guidelines Advisory Committee Scientific Report to the Secretary of Health and Human Services*. Updated August 24, 2021. Accessed July 13, 2023. https://health.gov/sites/default/files/2019-09/10_F-4_Cancer_Prevention.pdf

55. National Cancer Institute. *Obesity and Cancer Fact Sheet*. Published March 2, 2017. Accessed July 13, 2023. https://www.cancer.gov/about-cancer/causes-prevention/risk/obesity/obesity-fact-sheet

56. Kojima Y, Volkmer J-P, McKenna K, et al. CD47-blocking antibodies restore phagocytosis and prevent atherosclerosis. *Nature*. 2016;536:86–90.

57. Folkman J. Tumor angiogenesis: therapeutic implications. *N Engl J Med*. 1971;285(21):1182–1186.

58. National Cancer Institute. Angiogenesis inhibitors. Updated April 2, 2018. Accessed July 13, 2023. https://www.cancer.gov/about-cancer/treatment/types/immunotherapy/angiogenesis-inhibitors-fact-sheet

59. Moulton KS, Heller E, Konerding MA, Flynn E, Palinski W, Folkman J. Angiogenesis inhibitors endostatin or TNP-470 reduce intimal neovascularization and plaque growth in apolipoprotein E–deficient mice. *Circulation*. 1999;(13):1726–1732.

60. Libby P, Sidlow R, Lin AE, et al. Clonal hematopoiesis: crossroads of aging, cardiovascular disease, and cancer: JACC review topic of the week. *J Am Coll Cardiol*. 2019;74(4):567–577.

61. Modell B, Khan M, Darlison M, Westwood MA, Ingram D, Pennell DJ. Improved survival of thalassaemia major in the UK and relation to T2* cardiovascular magnetic resonance. *J Cardiovasc Magn Reson*. 2008;10(1):42.

62. Cunningham CH, Arai T, Yang PC, McConnell MV, Pauly JM, Conolly SM. Positive contrast magnetic resonance imaging of cells labeled with magnetic nanoparticles. *Magn Reson Med*. 2005;53(5):999–1005.

63. Terashima M, Uchida M, Kosuge H, et al. Human ferritin cages for imaging vascular macrophages. *Biomaterials*. 2011;32(5):1430–1437.

64. Branham M. How and why do fireflies light up? *Scientific American*. September 5, 2005. Accessed July 13, 2023. https://www.scientificamerican.com/article/how-and-why-do-fireflies/

65. Terashima M, Ehara S, Yang E, et al. In vivo bioluminescence imaging of inducible nitric oxide synthase gene expression in vascular inflammation. *Mol Imaging Biol*. 2011;13(6):1061–1066.

66. Rogers IS, Nasir K, Figueroa AL, et al. Feasibility of FDG imaging of the coronary arteries: comparison between acute coronary syndrome and stable angina. *JACC Cardiovasc Imaging*. 2010;3(4):388–397.

67. Zaman RT, Kosuge H, Pratx G, Carpenter C, Xing L, McConnell MV. Fiber-optic system for dual-modality imaging of glucose probes 18F-FDG and 6-NBDG in atherosclerotic plaques. *PLoS One*. 2014;9:e108108.

68. Amsallem M, Saito T, Tada Y, Dash R, McConnell MV. Magnetic resonance imaging and positron emission tomography approaches to imaging vascular and cardiac inflammation. *Circ J*. 2016;80(6):1269–1277.

69. Zaman RT, Yousefi S, Chibana H, et al. In vivo translation of the CIRPI system: revealing molecular pathology of rabbit aortic atherosclerotic plaques. *J Nucl Med*. 2019;60(9):1308–1316.

70. Farquhar JW, Maccoby N, Wood PD, et al. Community education for cardiovascular health. *Lancet*. 1977;1(8023):1192–1195.

71. Eapen ZJ, Turakhia MP, McConnell MV, et al. Defining a mobile health roadmap for cardiovascular health and disease. *J Am Heart Assoc*. 2016; 5(7):e003119.

72. Stanford Medicine. MyHeart Counts and My Fitness Counts. Accessed July 13, 2023. https://med.stanford.edu/myheartcounts.html

73. McConnell MV, Shcherbina A, Pavlovic A, et al. Feasibility of obtaining measures of lifestyle from a smartphone app: the MyHeart Counts cardiovascular health study. *JAMA Cardiol*. 2017;2(1):67–76.

74. Topol EJ. *The Patient Will See You Now: The Future of Medicine Is in Your Hands*. Basic Books; 2016.

75. American Heart Association. Life's Essential 8. Accessed July 13, 2023. https://www.heart.org/en/healthy-living/healthy-lifestyle/lifes-essential-8

76. American Cancer Society. Cancer Risk and Prevention. Accessed July 13, 2023. https://www.cancer.org/cancer/risk-prevention.html

77. Lloyd-Jones DM, Hong Y, Labarthe D, et al. Defining and setting national goals for cardiovascular health promotion and disease reduction: the American Heart Association's strategic Impact Goal through 2020 and beyond. *Circulation*. 2010;121(4):586–613.

78. Moore SC, Patel AV, Matthews CE, et al. Leisure time physical activity of moderate to vigorous intensity and mortality: a large pooled cohort analysis. *PLoS Med*. 2012;9:e1001335.

79. Physical Activity Guidelines Advisory Committee. *2018 Physical Activity Guidelines Advisory Committee Scientific Report to the Secretary of Health and Human Services*. Updated August 24, 2021. Accessed July 13, 2023. https://health.gov/paguidelines/second-edition/report.aspx

80. Office of Disease Prevention and Health Promotion, US Department of Health and Human Services. *Physical Activity Guidelines for Americans, 2nd edition.* Published 2018. Accessed July 13, 2023. https://health.gov /sites/default/files/2019-09/Physical_Activity_Guidelines_2nd_edition .pdf

81. McConnell MV. The new Google Fit helps make your heart points count. Published August 21, 2018. Accessed July 13, 2023. https://blog.verily.com /2018/08/the-new-google-fit-helps-make-your.html

82. Huang H, Yan Z, Chen Y, Liu F. A social contagious model of the obesity epidemic. *Sci Rep.* 2016;6:37961.

83. Stanford University. Health by stealth. Accessed July 13, 2023. https://125 .stanford.edu/health-by-stealth/

84. Zacharia J. The Bing "Marshmallow Studies": 50 years of continuing research. Published September 24, 2015. Accessed July 13, 2023. https:// bingschool.stanford.edu/news/bing-marshmallow-studies-50-years -continuing-research

85. Pollan M. *Food Rules: An Eater's Manual.* Penguin Books; 2009.

86. Sacks FM, Lichtenstein AH, Wu JHY, et al. Dietary fats and cardiovascular disease: a presidential advisory from the American Heart Association. *Circulation.* 2017;136(3):e1–e23.

87. de Cabo R, Mattson MP. Effects of intermittent fasting on health, aging, and disease. *N Engl J Med.* 2019;381:2541–2551.

88. Liu D, Huang Y, Huang C, et al. Calorie restriction with or without time-restricted eating in weight loss. *N Engl J Med.* 2022;386:1495–1504.

89. Wang M, Wang Z, Lee Y, et al. Dietary meat, trimethylamine N-oxide-related metabolites, and incident cardiovascular disease among older adults: the Cardiovascular Health Study. *Arterioscler Thromb Vasc Biol.* 2022;42: e273–e288.

90. Witkowski M, Weeks TL, Hazen SL. Gut microbiota and cardiovascular disease. *Circ Res.* 2020;127(4):553–570.

91. Gardner CD, Landry MJ, Perelman D, et al. Effect of a ketogenic diet versus Mediterranean diet on glycated hemoglobin in individuals with pre-diabetes and type 2 diabetes mellitus: The interventional Keto-Med randomized crossover trial. *Am J Clin Nutr.* 2022;116(3):640–652.

92. American Heart Association. *Life's Essential 8—How to Eat Better Fact Sheet.* Accessed July 13, 2023. https://www.heart.org/en/healthy-living /healthy-lifestyle/lifes-essential-8/how-to-eat-better-fact-sheet

93. Agatston A. *The South Beach Diet: The Delicious, Doctor-Designed Foolproof Plan for Fast and Healthy Weight Loss.* St. Martins Paperback; 2003.

94. Rosen CJ, Ingelfinger JR. Shifting tides offer new hope for obesity. *N Engl J Med.* 2022;387:271–273.

95. American Heart Association. The ugly truth about vaping. Accessed July 13, 2023. https://www.heart.org/en/healthy-living/healthy-lifestyle/quit-smoking-tobacco/the-ugly-truth-about-vaping

96. Weintraub K. Sleep vs. exercise? *New York Times.* December 8, 2017. Accessed July 13, 2023. https://www.nytimes.com/2017/12/08/well/sleep-vs-exercise.html

97. Rosenberger ME, Buman MP, Haskell WL, McConnell MV, Carstensen LL. Twenty-four hours of sleep, sedentary behavior, and physical activity with nine wearable devices. *Med Sci Sports Exerc.* 2016;48(3):457–465.

98. McConnell MV, Vavouranakis I, Wu LL, Vaughan DE, Ridker PM. Effects of a single, daily alcoholic beverage on lipid and hemostatic markers of cardiovascular risk. *Am J Cardiol.* 1997;80(9):1226–1228.

99. Lankester J, Zanetti D, Ingelsson E, Assimes TL. Alcohol use and cardiometabolic risk in the UK Biobank: a Mendelian randomization study. *PLoS One.* 2021;16(8):e0255801.

100. American Cancer Society. *American Cancer Society Guideline for Diet and Physical Activity for Cancer Prevention.* Published June 9, 2020. Accessed July 13, 2023. https://www.cancer.org/cancer/risk-prevention/diet-physical-activity/acs-guidelines-nutrition-physical-activity-cancer-prevention.html

101. Isath A, Kanwal A, Virk HUH, et al. The effect of yoga on cardiovascular disease risk factors: a meta-analysis. *Curr Probl Cardiol.* 2023;48(5):101593.

102. Levine GN, Allen K, Braun LT, et al. Pet ownership and cardiovascular risk: a scientific statement from the American Heart Association. *Circulation.* 2013;127(23):2353–2363.

103. Stanford Health Care. *Taking Care of My Heart—Dr. Michael McConnell.* YouTube. February 7, 2011. Accessed July 13, 2023. https://www.youtube.com/watch?v=kXURxpy5SMg

104. American Heart Association. Healthy bond for life. Accessed July 13, 2023. https://www.heart.org/en/healthy-living/healthy-bond-for-life-pets

105. Knowles JW, Zarafshar S, Pavlovic A, et al. Impact of a genetic risk score for coronary artery disease on reducing cardiovascular risk: a pilot randomized controlled study. *Front Cardiovasc Med.* 2017;4:53.

106. Family Heart Foundation. Familial hypercholesterolemia. Accessed July 13, 2023. https://thefhfoundation.org/

107. American College of Cardiology. Mobile and web apps. Accessed July 13, 2023. https://www.acc.org/Tools-and-Practice-Support/Mobile-Resources

108. Arnett DK, Blumenthal RS, Albert MA, et al. 2019 ACC/AHA guideline on the primary prevention of cardiovascular disease: a report of the Amer-

ican College of Cardiology/American Heart Association Task Force on Clinical Practice Guidelines. *Circulation*. 2019;140(11):e596–e646.

109. Centers for Disease Control and Prevention. Get a cholesterol test. Published September 8, 2020. Accessed July 13, 2023. https://www.cdc.gov /cholesterol/cholesterol_screening.htm

110. MedlinePlus. Cholesterol levels: what you need to know. Updated October 2, 2020. Accessed July 13, 2023. https://medlineplus.gov/cholesterolle velswhatyouneedtoknow.html

111. Sniderman AD, Navar AM, Thanassoulis G. Apolipoprotein B vs low-density lipoprotein cholesterol and non-high-density lipoprotein cholesterol as the primary measure of apolipoprotein B lipoprotein-related risk: the debate is over. *JAMA Cardiol*. 2022;7(3):257–258.

112. Flynn JT, Kaelber DC, Baker-Smith CM, et al. Clinical practice guideline for screening and management of high blood pressure in children and adolescents. *Pediatrics*. 2017;140(3):e20171904.

113. American Heart Association. High Blood Pressure. Accessed July 13, 2023. https://www.heart.org/en/health-topics/high-blood-pressure

114. Omron Healthcare, Inc. Wearable blood pressure monitor & watch. Accessed July 13, 2023. https://omronhealthcare.com/products/heartguide -wearable-blood-pressure-monitor-bp8000m/

115. American Diabetes Association. Diagnosis. Accessed July 13, 2023. https:// diabetes.org/diabetes/a1c/diagnosis

116. Centers for Disease Control and Prevention. Prediabetes—your chance to prevent type 2 diabetes. Published June 11, 2020. Accessed July 13, 2023. https://www.cdc.gov/diabetes/basics/prediabetes.html

117. Zahedani AD, Torbaghan SS, Rahili S, et al. Improvement in glucose regulation using a digital tracker and continuous glucose monitoring in healthy adults and those with type 2 diabetes. *Diabetes Ther*. 2021;12(7): 1871–1886.

118. Cainzos-Achirica M, Di Carlo PA, Handy CE, et al. Coronary artery calcium score: the "mammogram" of the heart? *Curr Cardiol Rep*. 2018;20(9):70.

119. Multi-Ethnic Study of Atherosclerosis (MESA). Accessed July 13, 2023. https://www.mesa-nhlbi.org/Calcium/input.aspx

120. Verily Project Baseline. Cardiologist Q&A: researching a new risk factor for heart disease. Accessed October 3, 2020. https://web.archive.org/web /20210724015425/https://blog.projectbaseline.com/2019/06/cardiologist -q-researching-new-risk.html

121. Yeboah J, McClelland RL, Polonsky TS, et al. Comparison of novel risk markers for improvement in cardiovascular risk assessment in intermediate-risk individuals. *JAMA*. 2012;308(8):788–795.

122. Quispe R, Al-Rifai M, Di Carlo PA, et al. Breast arterial calcium: a game changer in women's cardiovascular health? *JACC Cardiovasc Imaging.* 2019;12(12):2538–2548.

123. Ravenel JG, Nance JW. Coronary artery calcification in lung cancer screening. *Transl Lung Cancer Res.* 2018;7(3):361–367.

124. Ruparel M, Quaife SL, Dickson JL, et al. Evaluation of cardiovascular risk in a lung cancer screening cohort. *Thorax.* 2019;74(12):1140–1146.

125. Handy CE, Quispe R, Pinto X, et al. Synergistic opportunities in the interplay between cancer screening and cardiovascular disease risk assessment. *Circulation.* 2018;138(7):727–734.

126. Google. Diagnosing diabetic retinopathy with machine learning. Accessed October 16, 2022. https://about.google/stories/seeingpotential/

127. Poplin R, Varadarajan AV, Blumer K, et al. Prediction of cardiovascular risk factors from retinal fundus photographs via deep learning. *Nat Biomed Eng.* 2018;2:158–164.

128. McConnell, MV. Eyes: a window into heart health. Published February 19, 2018. Accessed July 13, 2023. https://blog.verily.com/2018/02/eyes-window-into-heart-health.html

129. Goldstein JL, Brown MS. A century of cholesterol and coronaries: from plaques to genes to statins. *Cell.* 2015;161(1):161–172.

130. Tahara N, Kai H, Ishibashi M, et al. Simvastatin attenuates plaque inflammation: evaluation by fluorodeoxyglucose positron emission tomography. *J Am Coll Cardiol.* 2006;48(9):1825–1831.

131. Hall SS. Genetics: a gene of rare effect. *Nature.* April 9, 2013. Accessed July 13, 2023. https://www.nature.com/articles/496152a

132. Raal FJ, Kallend D, Ray KK, et al. Inclisiran for the treatment of heterozygous familial hypercholesterolemia. *N Engl J Med.* 2020;382:1520–1530.

133. Visseren FLJ, Mach F, Smulders YM, et al. 2021 ESC Guidelines on cardiovascular disease prevention in clinical practice. *Eur Heart J.* 2021;42(34):3227–3337.

134. Lloyd-Jones DM, Morris PB, Ballantyne CM, et al. 2022 ACC expert consensus decision pathway on the role of nonstatin therapies for LDL-cholesterol lowering in the management of atherosclerotic cardiovascular disease risk: a report of the American College of Cardiology Soultion Set Oversight Committee. *J Am Coll Cardiol.* 2022;80(14):1366–1418.

135. Singh RR, Denton KM. Renal denervation. *Hypertension.* 2018;72(3):528–536.

136. Ridker PM, Glynn RJ, Hennekens CH. C-reactive protein adds to the predictive value of total and HDL cholesterol in determining risk of first myocardial infarction. *Circulation.* 1998;97(20):2007–2011.

137. Ridker PM, Buring JE, Shih J, Matias M, Hennekens CH. Prospective study of C-reactive protein and the risk of future cardiovascular events among apparently healthy women. *Circulation.* 1998;98(8):731–733.

138. Ridker PM, Danielson E, Fonseca FAH, et al. Rosuvastatin to prevent vascular events in men and women with elevated C-reactive protein. *N Engl J Med.* 2008;359:2195–2207.

139. Sherer Y, Shoenfeld Y. Mechanisms of disease: atherosclerosis in autoimmune diseases. *Nat Clin Pract Rheumatol.* 2006;2:99–106.

140. Bahrami H, Budoff M, Haberlen SA, et al. Inflammatory markers associated with subclinical coronary artery disease: the Multicenter AIDS Cohort Study. *J Am Heart Assoc.* 2016;5(6):e003371.

141. Ridker PM, Everett BM, Pradhan A, et al. Low-dose methotrexate for the prevention of atherosclerotic events. *N Engl J Med.* 2019;380: 752–762.

142. Tardif J-C, Kouz S, Waters DD, et al. Efficacy and safety of low-dose colchicine after myocardial infarction. *N Engl J Med.* 2019;381(26): 2497–2505.

143. Dhorepatil A, Ball S, Ghosh RK, Kondapaneni M, Lavie CJ. Canakinumab: promises and future in cardiometabolic diseases and malignancy. *Am J Med.* 2019;132(3):312–324.

144. Kosuge H, Sherlock SP, Kitagawa T, et al. Near infrared imaging and photothermal ablation of vascular inflammation using single-walled carbon nanotubes. *J Am Heart Assoc.* 2012;1(6):e002568.

145. Flores AM, Hosseini-Nassab N, Jarr K-U, et al. Pro-efferocytic nanoparticles are specifically taken up by lesional macrophages and prevent atherosclerosis. *Nat Nanotechnol.* 2020;15:154–161.

146. Jarr K-U, Nakamoto R, Doan BH, et al. Effect of CD47 blockade on vascular inflammation. *N Engl J Med.* 2021;384:382–383.

147. Lupu I-E, De Val S, Smart N. Coronary vessel formation in development and disease: mechanisms and insights for therapy. *Nat Rev Cardiol.* 2020; 17:790–806.

148. Maurea N, Coppola C, Piscopo G, et al. Pathophysiology of cardiotoxicity from target therapy and angiogenesis inhibitors. *J Cardiovasc Med.* 2016; 17(Suppl 1):S19–26.

149. Winter PM, Caruthers SD, Zhang H, Williams TA, Wickline SA, Lanza GM. Antiangiogenic synergism of integrin-targeted fumagillin nanoparticles and atorvastatin in atherosclerosis. *JACC Cardiovasc Imaging.* 2008; 1(5):624–634.

150. Van Craeyveld E, Jacobs F, Gordts SC, De Geest B. Gene therapy for familial hypercholesterolemia. *Curr Pharm Des.* 2011;17(24):2575–2591.

151. Verve Therapeutics. Verve Therapeutics doses first human with an investigational in vivo base editing medicine, VERVE-101, as a potential treatment for heterozygous familial hypercholesterolemia. Published July 12, 2022. Accessed July 13, 2023. https://ir.vervetx.com/news-releases/news-release-details/verve-therapeutics-doses-first-human-investigational-vivo-base

152. Steering Committee of the Physicians' Health Study Research Group. Final report on the aspirin component of the ongoing Physicians' Health Study. *N Engl J Med*. 1989;321(3):129–135.

153. US Preventive Services Task Force. Aspirin use to prevent cardiovascular disease: preventive medication. Published April 26, 2022. Accessed July 13, 2023. https://www.uspreventiveservicestaskforce.org/uspstf/recommendation/aspirin-to-prevent-cardiovascular-disease-preventive-medication

154. Maron DJ, Hochman JS, Reynolds HR, et al. Initial invasive or conservative strategy for stable coronary disease. *N Engl J Med*. 2020;382(15):1395–1407.

155. Warraich H. *State of the Heart: Exploring the History, Science, and Future of Cardiac Disease*. St. Martin's Publishing Group; 2019.

156. Chow EJ, Chen Y, Armstrong GT, et al. Underdiagnosis and undertreatment of modifiable cardiovascular risk factors among survivors of childhood cancer. *J Am Heart Assoc*. 2022;11(12):e024735.

157. Chuquin D, Abbate A, Bottinor W. Hypertension in cancer survivors: a review of the literature and suggested approach to diagnosis and treatment. *J Cardiovasc Pharmacol*. 2022;80(4):522–530.

158. Antman EM, Benjamin EJ, Harrington RA, et al. Acquisition, analysis, and sharing of data in 2015 and beyond: a survey of the landscape: a conference report from the American Heart Association Data Summit 2015. *J Am Heart Assoc*. 2015;4(11):e002810.

159. Rumsfeld JS, Joynt KE, Maddox TM. Big data analytics to improve cardiovascular care: promise and challenges. *Nat Rev Cardiol*. 2016;13(6):350–359.

160. Porter J, Boyd C, Skandari MR, Laiteerapong N. Revisiting the time needed to provide adult primary care. *J Gen Intern Med*. 2023;38(1):147–155.

161. American National Standards Institute, Consumer Technology Association. *Best Practices for Consumer Cardiovascular Technology Solutions (ANSI/CTA-2105)*. Published January 2022.

162. Bayoumy K, Gaber M, Elshafeey A, et al. Smart wearable devices in cardiovascular care: where we are and how to move forward. *Nat Rev Cardiol*. 2021;18:581–599.

163. Ferguson T, Olds T, Curtis R, et al. Effectiveness of wearable activity trackers to increase physical activity and improve health: a systematic review of systematic reviews and meta-analyses. *Lancet Digit Health*. 2022;4(8): e615–e626.

164. Zhou B, Perel P, Mensah GA, Ezzati M. Global epidemiology, health burden and effective interventions for elevated blood pressure and hypertension. *Nat Rev Cardiol*. 2021;18:785–802.

165. Chen LY, Tee BC-K, Chortos AL, et al. Continuous wireless pressure monitoring and mapping with ultra-small passive sensors for health monitoring and critical care. *Nat Commun*. 2014;5:5028.

166. PyrAmes Health. Blood pressure monitors. 2022. Accessed July 13, 2023. https://pyrameshealth.com/

167. Knowler WC, Barrett-Connor E, Fowler SE, et al. Reduction in the incidence of type 2 diabetes with lifestyle intervention or metformin. *N Engl J Med*. 2002;346(6):393–403.

168. Omada Health, Inc. Behavior change + integrated care, delivered at scale. Accessed July 13, 2023. https://www.omadahealth.com/platform

169. Kario K, Harada N, Okura A. Digital therapeutics in hypertension: evidence and perspectives. *Hypertension*. 2022;79(10):2148–2158.

170. Gazit T, Gutman M, Beatty AL. Assessment of hypertension control among adults participating in a mobile technology blood pressure self-management program. *JAMA Netw Open*. 2021;4(10):e2127008.

171. Ang A. Japan clears CureApp's DTx app for hypertension. *MobiHealthNews*. May 8, 2022. Accessed July 13, 2023. https://www.mobihealthnews .com/news/asia/japan-clears-cureapps-dtx-app-hypertension

172. Diabetes Prevention Program Outcomes Study Research Group; Orchard TJ, Temprosa M, et al. Long-term effects of the Diabetes Prevention Program interventions on cardiovascular risk factors: a report from the DPP Outcomes Study. *Diabet Med*. 2013;30(1):46–55.

173. Thamman R, Janardhanan R. Cardiac rehabilitation using telemedicine: the need for tele cardiac rehabilitation. *Rev Cardiovasc Med*. 2020;21(4): 497–500.

174. Egbedi H. Moving Analytics: A disruptive telehealth innovation for patients with cardiovascular diseases. *Ventures Africa*. November 15, 2016. Accessed July 13, 2023. https://venturesafrica.com/features/moving-analytics -a-disruptive-telehealth-innovation-for-patients-with-cardiovascular -diseases/

175. Funahashi T, Boro L, Joshi N. Saving lives with virtual cardiac rehab. *NEJM Catalyst*. Published August 28, 2019. Accessed July 13, 2023. https://catalyst .nejm.org/saving-lives-virtual-cardiac-rehab/

176. Thomas RJ, Beatty AL, Beckie TM, et al. Home-based cardiac rehabilitation: a scientific statement from the American Association of Cardiovascular and Pulmonary Rehabilitation, the American Heart Association, and the American College of Cardiology. *Circulation*. 2019;140:e69–e89.

177. Bell AG. The History and Mystery of Eliza. *CoRecursive Podcast*. Published July 5, 2022. Accessed July 13, 2023. https://corecursive.com/eliza-with-jeff-shrager/#

178. Malloy T. Mayo researchers use AI to detect weak heart pump via patients' Apple Watch ECGs. *Mayo Clinic News Network*. May 2, 2022. Accessed July 13, 2023. https://newsnetwork.mayoclinic.org/discussion/mayo-researchers-use-ai-to-detect-weak-heart-pump-via-patients-apple-watch-ecgs/

179. Yao X, Rushlow DR, Inselman JW, et al. Artificial intelligence-enabled electrocardiograms for identification of patients with low ejection fraction: a pragmatic, randomized clinical trial. *Nat Med*. 2021;27(5): 815–819.

180. Eko Devices, Inc. FDA grants "breakthrough" designation to Eko's ECG-based low ejection fraction screening algorithm, designed to improve detection of heart failure. *GlobeNewswire*. December 18, 2019. Accessed July 13, 2023. https://www.globenewswire.com/news-release/2019/12/18/1962218/0/en/FDA-Grants-Breakthrough-Designation-to-Eko-s-ECG-based-Low-Ejection-Fraction-Screening-Algorithm-Designed-to-Improve-Detection-of-Heart-Failure.html

181. Volpara Health. Volpara Health collaborates with Microsoft to accelerate the research and development of software that uses mammograms to identify potential cardiovascular issues. Published August 4, 2022. Accessed July 13, 2023. https://www.volparahealth.com/news/volpara-health-collaborates-with-microsoft-to-accelerate-the-research-and-development-of-software-that-uses-mammograms-to-identify-potential-cardiovascular-issues/

182. iCAD Inc. iCAD and Solis Mammography ink deal to collaborate on use of AI to evaluate risk of cardiovascular disease. *GlobeNewswire*. October 11, 2022. Accessed July 13, 2023. https://www.globenewswire.com/news-release/2022/10/11/2531784/0/en/iCAD-and-Solis-Mammography-Ink-Deal-to-Collaborate-on-Use-of-AI-to-Evaluate-Risk-of-Cardiovascular-Disease.html

183. Topol E. *Deep Medicine: How Artificial Intelligence Can Make Healthcare Human Again*. Hachette UK; 2019.

184. Editors; Rubin E. Striving for diversity in research studies. *N Engl J Med*. 2021;385:1429–1430.

185. Lim JI, Regillo CD, Sadda SR, et al. Artificial intelligence detection of diabetic retinopathy: subgroup comparison of the EyeArt System with ophthalmologists' dilated exams. *Ophthalmol Sci.* 2022;3(1):100228.

186. Parakh K, Dirksen A. *Searching for Health: The Smart Way to Find Information Online and Put It to Use.* Johns Hopkins University Press; 2021.

187. Kelly SM. Google begins rolling out its ChatGPT rival. *CNN Business.* March 21, 2023. Accessed July 13, 2023. https://www.cnn.com/2023/03/21/tech/google-bard/index.html

188. American Lung Association. *Tobacco Trends Brief.* Accessed July 13, 2023. https://www.lung.org/research/trends-in-lung-disease/tobacco-trends-brief/overall-tobacco-trends

189. US Food & Drug Administration. FDA announces plans for proposed rule to reduce addictiveness of cigarettes and other combusted tobacco products. *FDA News Release.* June 21, 2022. Accessed July 13, 2023. https://www.fda.gov/news-events/press-announcements/fda-announces-plans-proposed-rule-reduce-addictiveness-cigarettes-and-other-combusted-tobacco

190. Greger M. How Not to Die: Preventing and Treating Disease with Diet. Food Is Medicine Conference, December 19, 2022. Accessed July 13, 2023. https://www.youtube.com/watch?v=uiPWPpmrwF8

191. The Annie E. Casey Foundation. Exploring America's food deserts. Published February 13, 2021. Accessed July 13, 2023. https://www.aecf.org/blog/exploring-americas-food-deserts

192. Geisinger Health. Fresh Food Farmacy. Accessed July 13, 2023. https://www.geisinger.org/freshfoodfarmacy

193. Mozaffarian D, Blanck HM, Garfield KM, Wassung A, Petersen R. A Food is Medicine approach to achieve nutrition security and improve health. *Nat Med.* 2022;28:2238–2240.

194. Fleischhacker SE, Woteki CE, Coates PM, et al. Strengthening national nutrition research: rationale and options for a new coordinated federal research effort and authority. *Am J Clin Nutr.* 2020;112(3):721–769.

195. American Heart Association. Statement by Dr. Rajiv J. Shah, president of The Rockefeller Foundation, and Nancy Brown, CEO of the American Heart Association, on new Food Is Medicine research initiative. Published September 28, 2022. Accessed July 13, 2023. https://newsroom.heart.org/news/statement-by-dr-rajiv-j-shah-president-of-the-rockefeller-foundation-and-nancy-brown-ceo-of-the-american-heart-association-on-new-food-is-medicine-research-initiative

196. Althoff T, Sosič R, Hicks JL, King AC, Delp SL, Leskovec J. Large-scale physical activity data reveal worldwide activity inequality. *Nature.* 2017; 547:336–339.

197. King AC, Winter SJ, Sheats JL, et al. Leveraging citizen science and information technology for population physical activity promotion. *Transl J Am Coll Sports Med.* 2016;1(4):30–44.

198. Stanford Medicine. Our voice: citizen science for health equity. Accessed July 13, 2023. https://med.stanford.edu/ourvoice.html

199. American Heart Association. 2024 Health equity impact goal. Accessed July 13, 2023. https://www.heart.org/en/about-us/2024-health-equity-impact-goal

200. The RURAL Cohort Study. Accessed July 13, 2023. https://www.theruralstudy.org/

201. The RURAL Cohort Study—Mobile Examination Unit. Accessed July 13, 2023. https://youtu.be/KYzF5kZck3s

202. Abnousi F. Connecting people with health resources. Meta. Published October 28, 2019. Accessed July 13, 2023. https://about.fb.com/news/2019/10/connecting-people-with-health-resources/

203. Sim I. Mobile devices and health. *N Engl J Med.* 2019;381(10):956–968.

204. CommonHealth. Manage your health data. Accessed July 13, 2023. https://www.commonhealth.org/

205. Google Health. Participate in health studies. Accessed July 13, 2023. https://health.google/consumers/health-studies/

206. American College of Cardiology. ASCVD Risk Estimator Plus Resources. Accessed July 13, 2023. https://tools.acc.org/ascvd-risk-estimator-plus/#!/content/resources/

207. Patel AP, Wang M, Kartoun U, Ng K, Khera AV. Quantifying and understanding the higher risk of atherosclerotic cardiovascular disease among South Asian individuals: results from the UK Biobank Prospective Cohort Study. *Circulation.* 2021;144(6):410–422.

208. Dzaye O, Razavi AC, Dardari ZA, et al. Modeling the recommended age for initiating coronary artery calcium testing among at-risk young adults. *J Am Coll Cardiol.* 2021;78(16):1573–1583.

209. Gidding SS, Wiegman A, Groselj U, et al. Paediatric familial hypercholesterolaemia screening in Europe—public policy background and recommendations. *Eur J Prev Cardiol.* 2022;29(18):2301–2311.

210. Luirink IK, Wiegman A, Kusters DM, et al. 20-year follow-up of statins in children with familial hypercholesterolemia. *N Engl J Med.* 2019;381:1547–1556.

211. Gregory EF, Miller JM, Wasserman RC, et al. Adherence to pediatric universal cholesterol testing guidelines across body mass index categories: A CER2 Cohort Study. *Circ Cardiovasc Qual Outcomes.* 2020;13(8):e006519.

212. Real Sports with Bryant Gumbel. *Chris Evert Interview*. Facebook video. June 21, 2022. Accessed July 13, 2023. https://www.facebook.com/real sportshbo/videos/760564578313449/

213. Akbari MR, Gojska N, Narod SA. Coming of age in Canada: a study of population-based genetic testing for breast and ovarian cancer. *Curr Oncol*. 2017;24(5):282–283.

214. identifeye HEALTH. The broad lens: health you can see. Accessed July 13, 2023. https://www.identifeye.health/

215. Centers for Disease Control and Prevention. *Diabetic Retinopathy*. Accessed July 13, 2023. https://www.cdc.gov/visionhealth/pdf/factsheet.pdf

216. US Food and Drug Administration. FDA permits marketing of artificial intelligence-based device to detect certain diabetes-related eye problems. *FDA News Release*. April 11, 2018. Accessed July 13, 2023. https://www.fda .gov/news-events/press-announcements/fda-permits-marketing -artificial-intelligence-based-device-detect-certain-diabetes-related-eye

217. Hickam JB, Frayser R. Studies of the retinal circulation in man. Observations on vessel diameter, arteriovenous oxygen difference, and mean circulation time. *Circulation*. 1966;33(2):302–316.

218. Seidelmann SB, Claggett B, Bravo PE, et al. Retinal vessel calibers in predicting long-term cardiovascular outcomes: the Atherosclerosis Risk in Communities Study. *Circulation*. 2016;134(18):1328–1338.

219. Chandra A, Seidelmann SB, Claggett BL, et al. The association of retinal vessel calibres with heart failure and long-term alterations in cardiac structure and function: the Atherosclerosis Risk in Communities Study. *Eur J Heart Fail*. 2019;21(10):1207–1215.

220. Zekavat SM, Raghu VK, Trinder M, et al. Deep learning of the retina enables phenome- and genome-wide analyses of the microvasculature. *Circulation*. 2021;145(2):134–150.

221. Rim TH, Lee CJ, Tham YC, et al. Deep-learning-based cardiovascular risk stratification using coronary artery calcium scores predicted from retinal photographs. *Lancet Digit Health*. 2021;3(5):e306–e316.

222. Cheung CY, Biousse V, Keane PA, Schiffrin EL, Wong TY. Hypertensive eye disease. *Nat Rev Dis Primers*. 2022;8(1):14.

223. Xue C, Li C, Chen DN, et al. Five-year incidence of arterial hypertension predicted by retinal vessel analysis: the Tongren Cohort Study. *Invest Ophthalmol Vis Sci*. 2022;63:1160–1160.

224. Kirollos S, Skilton M, Patel S, Arnott C. A systematic review of vascular structure and function in pre-eclampsia: non-invasive assessment and mechanistic links. *Front Cardiovasc Med*. 2019;6:166.

225. Wagner SK, Fu DJ, Faes L, et al. Insights into systemic disease through retinal imaging-based oculomics. *Transl Vis Sci Technol.* 2020;9(2):6.

226. Nusinovici S, Rim TH, Yu M, et al. Retinal photograph-based deep learning predicts biological age, and stratifies morbidity and mortality risk. *Age Ageing.* 2022;51(4):afac065.

227. Rajalakshmi R, Arulmalar S, Usha M, et al. Validation of smartphone based retinal photography for diabetic retinopathy screening. *PLoS One.* 2015; 10(9):e0138285.

228. Mehta A, Vasquez N, Ayers CR, et al. Independent association of lipoprotein(a) and coronary artery calcification with atherosclerotic cardiovascular risk. *J Am Coll Cardiol.* 2022;79(8):757–768.

229. Office of the Assistant Secretary for Health. HHS Secretary Becerra appoints new national fitness foundation's board of directors. US Department of Health and Human Services. Published August 29, 2022. Accessed July 13, 2023. https://www.hhs.gov/about/news/2022/08/29/hhs-secretary-becerra-appoints-new-national-fitness-foundations-board-of-directors.html

230. Office of Disease Prevention and Health Promotion. Presidential Youth Fitness Program. Updated March 24, 2023. Accessed July 13, 2023. https://health.gov/our-work/nutrition-physical-activity/presidents-council/programs-awards/presidential-youth-fitness-program

231. Physical Activity Alliance. *The 2022 United States Report Card on Physical Activity for Children and Youth.* Published October 24, 2022. Accessed July 13, 2023. https://paamovewithus.org/news/2022-u-s-report-on-physical-activity-for-children-and-youth/

232. Richtel M. The income gap is becoming a physical-activity divide. *New York Times.* March 24, 2023. Accessed July 13, 2023. https://www.nytimes.com/2023/03/24/health/sports-physical-education-children.html

Index

24-hour cycle, 89, 172

access. *See* health equity
Active Zone Minutes, 142, 184
activity inequality, 160, 185
Agatston, Arthur, 87. *See also* diet
Agatston score, 87. *See also* coronary
   artery calcium
alcohol, 62, 79, 90–92, 96, 123
Alcoholics Anonymous, 90
Alexa. *See* chatbot
Alphazero, 149–50, 153
Alzheimer's disease, 180
American Academy of Pediatrics, 69,
   104
American Cancer Society (ACS), 78,
   79, 92, 158, 171
American College of Cardiology
   (ACC), 98, 122, 140, 148
American Heart Association (AHA),
   10, 5481, 148, 156–57, 159, 170,
   176; food programs, 87, 158–59;
   Go Red for Women campaign,
   49–50; guidances, 12–13, 74, 76,
   85, 87, 94, 98, 105, 122, 148, 156;
   Health Tech forum, 74; Life's
   Essential, 8, 72, 78–79, 89, 100,
   124, 171; Life's Simple, 7, 79, 171;

2020 Impact Goal, 79; 2024 Health
   Equity Goal, 161; 2030 Impact
   Goal, 10, 92, 160, 170, 187
Android, 164–65
aneurysm: aortic, 60, 143; abdominal
   aortic aneurysm (AAA), 60
angina. *See* chest pain
angiogenesis, 41–42, 64–68, 128–29
angiogram, 30–31, 42–45, 50, 111
angioplasty, 39, 45, 131
angiotensin, 123
aorta, 21–23, 29–30, 32, 33, 60, 143.
   See also aneurysm
apolipoprotein-B (apoB). *See*
   cholesterol
app(s), 98–99, 145, 148, 151, 160–61,
   167
Apple, 74, 142–43, 163–65. *See also*
   MyHeart Counts study
artificial intelligence (AI), 76, 106,
   113–14, 138–54, 161, 172,
   173–82
artificial pancreas. *See* glucose
aspirin, 130–31, 133, 135–36, 162
atheroma. *See* atherosclerosis
atherosclerosis: ASCVD Risk Score,
   75, 97–100, 114, 152, 163, 166–68,
   177–77, 181; atheroma, 15, 35–38,